SPIRITUAL CARE
The Nurse's Role

Judith Allen Shelly
& Sharon Fish

Third
Edition

INTERVARSITY PRESS
DOWNERS GROVE, ILLINOIS 60515

InterVarsity Press is the book-publishing division of InterVarsity Christian Fellowship, a student movement active on campus at hundreds of universities, colleges and schools of nursing. For information about local and regional activities, write Public Relations Dept., InterVarsity Christian Fellowship, 6400 Schroeder Rd., P.O. Box 7895, Madison, WI 53707-7895.

Distributed in Canada through InterVarsity Press, 860 Denison St., Unit 3, Markham, Ontario L3R 4H1, Canada.

The Scripture quotations contained herein, unless otherwise noted, are from the Revised Standard Version of the Bible copyrighted 1946, 1952, 1971 by the Division of Christian Education of the National Council of the Churches of Christ in the U.S.A. and are used by permission. All rights reserved.

ISBN 0-8308-1254-7

Printed in the United States of America

Library of Congress Cataloging in Publication Data is available.

17	16	15	14	13	12	11	10	9	8	7	6	5	4	3	2	1
99	98	97	96	95	94	93	92	91	90	89	88					

To Tressie

Tables

Figures

Foreword

Six years ago, the long-range plan of Nurses Christian Fellowship targeted 1978 for the publication of a text addressing the nurse's role in spiritual care. I thank God this publication achieves this goal. I vividly recall how as a faculty member I longed for references that would provide practical assistance for this important facet of nursing. *Spiritual Care: The Nurse's Role* provides a body of knowledge and techniques for nurses and other health-care workers so they can assist patients and their families in this area more effectively. The addition of a workbook makes it a double treat, enabling nurses or students to pursue independently this dimension of care in greater depth.

There is a history behind this publication. More than a decade ago, NCF staff, under the inspiration and leadership of Tressie Myers, endeavored to approach this area through seminars, workshops and by teaching spiritual care in classrooms at the invitation of faculty. Some of these early workshops were "Spiritual Needs of Patients" (Berkeley, 1966), "Spiritual Needs of the Dying Patient and His Family" (Seattle, 1967), "Is God on Your Nursing Team?" (Detroit, 1968) and "Spiritual Needs of Patients" (Chicago, 1968).

During 1968 a sampling of nurses, doctors, pastors and chaplains from across the country responded to questions asked to determine basic spiritual needs, how these are expressed in health and illness, and how to identify them. In the summer a double task force underwritten by funds from the Lilly Foundation met for a week to examine the data collected. One task force explored spiritual needs as a part of total patient care; the second pursued the Christian nurse's philosophy of nursing. This was a springboard to continuing work on these two topics by members of these committees and our staff.

The following summer the first group reconvened to process data collected from a pilot project on spiritual needs. (The results of this survey are found in appendix A of this text.) Findings indicated that patients were aware of their own spiritual needs and were willing to discuss them with nurse interviewers. A conclusion drawn from the study was that persistent and unresolved spiritual needs may affect the total body function and the patient's progress toward health. Nurses were seen as the key persons to pick up cues related to those needs. A nurse could be of direct help to the patient in personally offering spiritual assistance and for making referral to resource people.

This study triggered the need for greater depth in our workshops, more utilization of nursing faculty in teaching them and a broader challenge to the profession to implement these concepts. Helen McMurtry, then director of nursing education at Barnes Hospital School of Nursing in St. Louis, served on the National Advisory Committee for NCF and chaired the 1968-69 ad hoc committee which guided the summer projects. In 1970 she became the central area director for NCF and continued to spearhead these developments.

Ruth Stoll, on a year's special assignment with NCF, reviewed pertinent literature in nursing and pastoral counseling. She and Jean Stallwood Hess (who designed a conceptual model of man as a spiritual being) developed a workshop based on this research and the results of the pilot project. In 1972 they presented a four-day workshop in Chicago entitled "Persons in Crisis." This focused on man as a spiritual being, on needs in stress and crisis, and on the nurse's role in intervention. A forerunner of this, funded by a mental health grant, was held six months earlier in Louisville, cosponsored by Spaulding College and Nurses Christian Fellowship. A preliminary assignment for "Persons in Crisis" participants was to use an interview guide with one or two patients concerning their spiritual needs. The workshop was evaluated, refined and then held in California, Washington, Illinois, Ohio, Pennsylvania, New York and New Jersey over the next four years. Follow-up questionnaires, sent to three hundred fifty participants in 1976, indicated a continued excitement about the content which many had adapted for use clinically, in the classroom and for inservice education. Participants requested more specific guidelines for assessing and meeting patients' spiritual needs.

Believing the content that had been developed should be more broadly available to nurses, I asked Sharon Fish and Judy Shelly to write this book. God had prepared them for this assignment. "Man and His Needs in the Presence of Illness" was Sharon's master's thesis before she joined NCF staff. Judy interrupted her NCF employment to obtain a seminary education that included pastoral-care training. She worked as a hospital staff nurse during her two years at seminary. In this text and workbook they bring together research, theory and practice to give specific guidelines to help you define your responsibility in spiritual care. I am delighted with their product and wholeheartedly commend it to you as the launching pad for increasing your ability to assist patients spiritually and for your own spiritual growth. Happy reading and growing!

Grace Wallace
Director, Nurses Christian Fellowship
November 1977

Preface

"I don't even know what a spiritual need is. How am I supposed to meet it?"

If you think a spiritual need is a vague, undefinable entity that cannot be accurately assessed, much less met, this text is for you. *Spiritual Care: The Nurse's Role* attempts to define the spiritual dimension and make it a natural part of nursing practice that easily fits into the nursing process.

The text is liberally sprinkled with case studies. The majority are drawn from nursing experiences with medical-surgical patients in a large metropolitan hospital. We believe the principles of spiritual care apply to patients in a variety of settings. We hope that after reading this book you will have the desire to record your own interaction with patients who demonstrate spiritual needs. This could provide valuable information for the development of materials related to specific areas of nursing and patient populations not dealt with in this text, for example, spiritual needs of children.

Spiritual Care: The Nurse's Role is not meant to be read in isolation. *Spiritual Care Workbook,* also published by InterVarsity Press, accompanies it. The workbook, designed for both individual and small group use, consists of nine units which correspond with the chapters of this text. Nursing *faculty* will find the material in the text and workbook arranged for a semester course on the spiritual dimension of nursing. Or the material could be integrated into existing curricula. *Nurses and nursing students* may also use the text and workbook as an independent study project. The material is readily adaptable to *in-service or continuing education courses* in health-related facilities. The text and workbook also provide the basis for weekly or monthly *Nurses Christian Fellow-*

ship meetings. Finally, it is our hope that this book and the workbook are adaptable to a wide variety of *health-care workers* other than nurses, to *physicians,* to *hospital chaplains,* to *ministers* who visit hospitals and to all *those with visitation ministries.*

This book begins in chapters one and two by setting spiritual care in the context of nursing and of values. Chapter three defines spiritual needs while chapter four incorporates these into the nursing process. Chapters five through eight discuss four specific resources available to nurses for meeting spiritual needs of patients. The closing chapter introduces the spiritual resources available to nurses themselves.

One of our primary assertions throughout is that one's personal value system influences one's understanding of the nurse's role in spiritual care. This system of values is based on what one believes about the nature of God and man. The authors' system of values falls within the Judeo-Christian framework. We write from this perspective, believing the spiritual needs we have identified reflect the common humanity we all share regardless of race, creed or culture.

We have enjoyed writing this book and have learned much in the process. Our prayer is that as you read and study you will discover the spiritual dimension as the integrating force tying together the whole, promoting health and well-being in all areas of life, for yourself as well as for your patients.

Acknowledgments

The need for a text on spiritual care has been recognized for more than a decade. Data for it has been compiled over the years. Nurses Christian Fellowship's emphasis on helping nurses apply biblical principles to the care of patients enabled the ideas to grow and mature. We are indeed grateful to the following people who planted the seeds of the vision and nourished the concepts we have developed in this text:

Tressie Myers, Director of Nurses Christian Fellowship 1950-68, encouraged NCF to pioneer in the spiritual dimension of nursing.

Helen McMurtry, first in a voluntary capacity and later as central area director of Nurses Christian Fellowship, watered the vision and made it grow.

Jean Stallwood Hess, associate professor of nursing at Wayne State University, and Eleanor Flor Bretall, associate professor of nursing at University of Arizona, wrote up the initial spiritual needs research from which has sprouted many new shoots and is still stimulating both undergraduate and graduate research.

Jane Corwin Reeves, NCF staff member 1968-70 and 1972-73, and other staff pioneered in teaching spiritual needs in hospitals and schools of nursing.

Ruth Lichtenberger, Bonnie Meyer, Mary Thompson and Marge Rosti with Helen McMurtry comprised the task force for curriculum development which synthesized material being used in 1971 and developed a Curriculum Project Proposal targeted to present to the profession a body of knowledge relating to the spiritual dimension of man.

Ruth Stoll, associate professor of nursing at the University of Kentucky, was key developer of the "Persons in Crisis" workshops, and the faculty there taught nurses to more effectively meet patients' spiritual needs through these workshops.

Marilyne Gustafson, Melodie Chenevert, Judy Van Heukelem, Cindy Hall and Carol Chin read the original manuscript and gave many helpful suggestions.

Bill Bailey, John Boyle, Bill Showalter and George Ensworth, pastors who have contributed to our understanding of the use of prayer and Scripture with patients and the complementary roles of nurses and clergy.

Ellen Shelly typed and retyped for us, correcting errors along the way.

James Shelly, Judy Shelly's husband, our on-the-spot critic and encourager.

Claire Martin, Cherill Burrows and Jane Pomilio gave us permission to publish their 1976 research study on spiritual needs.

The faculty of Lutheran Theological Seminary at Philadelphia, the University of Rochester School of Nursing and Colgate Rochester Divinity School gave us the freedom and encouragement as graduate students to think through and develop the role of the nurse in spiritual care.

The Maclellen Foundation gave a generous grant to Nurses Christian Fellowship for materials development. And many kind individuals have also given to this work.

Grace Wallace, Director of Nurses Christian Fellowship, delegated to us the responsibility to develop these materials and has been our primary encourager.

Many NCF staff, students and graduate nurses over the years have contributed their ideas and shared their joys, struggles and visions with us.

Chapter 1
Responsible Nursing

Illness may precipitate a spiritual crisis. Since illness is man's reaction to disease, it is a time when men are brought face to face with the ultimate concerns of life.
Samuel Southard

People turn to God in times of crisis, and illness is among those times when people feel the need for spiritual guidance. Nurses, therefore, are in a unique position to bring spiritual aid to their patients and to the patients' families.
Margeurite Lucy Manfreda

By including assessment of spiritual needs along with assessment of the psychosocial and biological needs of patients, nurses can more effectively care for the whole person.
Jean Stallwood

Case 1. Mr. Richardson, age thirty-seven, was admitted to the hospital after a routine chest X ray revealed a small neoplasm on his right lung. The evening before surgery he was pacing up and down the corridor by his room. One of the staff nurses, observing his behavior, offered to sit and talk with him.

"You really appear concerned, Mr. Richardson," the nurse began.

"Guess I am," Mr. Richardson replied. "They're going to open me up tomorrow morning. The doctor said it might be cancer."

"You're probably feeling many things right now," responded the nurse.

"Yes," Mr. Richardson agreed, "and I guess I'm scared. I'm afraid I might not make it—that I might die on the operating table."

"What about death makes you afraid?" asked the nurse.

"Well," said Mr. Richardson, looking beyond the nurse and seeming to reflect for a moment. "To tell you the truth, I'm afraid of God. I feel guilty—like I don't measure up to his standards. I don't think I'm ready to meet God. Can you help me?" ■

Case 2. Mr. Conway, age forty-three, was admitted to a medical unit with a diagnosis of cirrhosis of the liver secondary to chronic alcoholism. Three weeks prior to admission Mr. Conway had been fired from his job as a security guard at a local manufacturing plant because of his failure to report regularly for duty. Immediately after he left the plant, his wife filed for divorce and moved out of the house along with their only child, a boy of fifteen.

Several days after his admission to the hospital, Mr. Conway began to verbalize his feelings to the nurse who was giving him evening care.

"Nurse, do you know what it's like to live this way?" Before the nurse could reply Mr. Conway went on. "My wife left me, you know. She couldn't take it any longer. I guess I should be able to understand that. But sometimes I get to wondering if God has given up on me. Does he really care or is he ready to wash his hands of me too?" ■

Case 3. Jennie Matthews, age twenty-three, was rushed to the emergency room following a three-car collision. Her parents were notified and came immediately to the hospital. The doctor took them aside and told them the news: Jennie's neck was broken. She had not regained consciousness. One nurse who was coming off duty brought the parents coffee and sat with them while they were waiting to see their daughter. Mr. Matthews turned to the nurse in tears. "Why? Why?" he pleaded. "Jennie's been such a good girl. She loved God . . . was going to be a missionary. Why did God let this happen to her?" ■

I don't think I'm ready to meet God. Can you help me? Does God really care about me, nurse? Why did God let this happen? If you had been the nurse in each of these situations, how would you have responded? Most of us would probably admit to feelings of inadequacy. We may be asking those same questions ourselves. How can we be expected to help others? Even if we could offer satisfactory answers, we would undoubtedly find communicating them no easy task.

The first course of action in situations like these might be to call for the hospital chaplain. This may be a legitimate decision. But a hospital chaplain is not always available, and even with the chaplain's therapeutic intervention, the nurse is the person most readily available when a patient needs to talk about his concerns, be they physical, emotional or spiritual. This fact should impress on us the necessity of becoming increasingly comfortable in dealing with the spiritual needs of patients and families who frequently look to us for support and encouragement. Spiritual care, briefly and basically defined, consists of assisting a person in establishing and/or maintaining a relationship with God. It is an integral part of responsible nursing.

Man, as individual women and men, is basically a religious creature; he seeks someone or something to worship. A Gallup poll conducted in 1975 reported that ninety-four per cent of the American people believed in God.[1] If each person polled had been asked, "What kind of a God do you believe in?" the answers would have varied greatly.

Some people, like Mr. Richardson, might describe God as a "resident policeman" who makes a person toe the line and fit in with certain heavenly standards that are humanly impossible to meet—a God to be feared. Others might see God as a benign and gentle father-figure whose only desire is that his children be happy all the time. Many people believe in a vague cosmic force that set the world in motion and then left it to spin on its own. This God may be thought to be responsible for the "acts of God" mentioned in insurance policies, and nothing more. Such a God is largely unknown and unknowable. He is certainly not a God who could meet the need for love and relationship Mr. Conway was expressing or a God who could give an acceptable answer to the parents of Jennie, who were searching for meaning and purpose in the face of tragedy.[2]

Nearly two thousand years ago a man named Paul stood up in the middle of a crowded marketplace in Greece and made an announcement to people who had incorporated an unknown god into their public worship. "Men of Athens," said Paul, "I perceive that in every way you are very religious. For as I passed along, and observed the objects of your worship, I found also an altar with this inscription, 'To an unknown god.' " (Acts 17:22-23).

Paul went on to say that the God they were worshiping as unknown was of an entirely different nature from the cold and impersonal gods of silver, gold and stone that covered the hillside. These other gods were humanly made. They were described several generations earlier in the Psalms (115:3-8) as having eyes that could not see, ears that could not hear and mouths that could not speak.

In contrast, the God Paul proclaimed was real and knowable. He was not a created god, but God the Creator, who made the world and everything in it. This God was not immobile. He could not be nailed to a pedestal, confined by space, time or the limits of human imagination. The "known God" was involved in the lives of men and women everywhere and able to satisfy all their needs. He was a personal God who actively sought after people, desiring that all come to know him intimately.[3]

A normal, healthy person is in control of his faculties and may seldom think about his need for a relationship with a personal God. He may even perceive himself to be a kind of god, believing that he is self-sufficient. In times of good health, life is active, full and in most ways predictable. Yet illness, suffering and death serve to remind us all that we are really not sufficient unto ourselves but are indeed very human and very helpless. The realization that, ultimately, we are not in control of our lives forces us to consider who is. If we conclude that God is in control, yet our God is largely unknown, we find ourselves in a fearful situation.

An "unknown god" can give little comfort to a suffering person. Only a God who is living and active and involved in the world can bring comfort and strength to a person overwhelmed with grief and wrestling with guilt, feelings of loneliness or the mystery of suffering. If an individual's religious training has not been meaningful and relevant to his life or if a person has become disillusioned about God through past experiences, God may appear as unknown, uncaring or even nonexistent. Illness may increase a person's feelings of alienation from God and precipitate a spiritual crisis.[4] Accurate assessment of spiritual needs and responsible nursing intervention can radically enrich the care of the whole person and thus facilitate healing. This example illustrates:

Case 4.   Mr. Levi was a sixty-five-year-old Jewish man with carcinoma of the bladder. He was frequently readmitted for cystoscopic examinations and transurethral resections for recurrent bladder tumors. He was consistently a "difficult patient." He screamed, moaned and cursed loudly when in pain and even when the pain subsided he remained demanding. Every medical and nursing measure was employed to relieve his constant bladder spasms but nothing seemed to work for very long. Finally one of the nurses decided to stay with him for a while after giving him his pain medication.

Mr. Levi began to relax after his injection and talk with the nurse. He began to reminisce about a recent trip to Israel. He had been deeply touched by seeing the places where the patriarchs had walked and the biblical battles had been fought. The nurse, reflecting Mr. Levi's awe, remarked, "God has always taken good care of his people." Mr. Levi grasped the nurse's hand tightly and wept. His pain diminished.

Within an hour Mr. Levi was again writhing in pain. It was too soon to repeat his pain medication. The nurse came in and put a hand on his shoulder. Mr. Levi relaxed slightly.

"I wish I could die!" exclaimed Mr. Levi. "The pain won't let up. I know it's not time for another shot. I know you can't do anything, nurse, but it's killing me."

"Mr. Levi," the nurse responded, "the only thing I can do is to pray and ask God to help you."

Mr. Levi responded positively to the nurse's suggestion and bowed his head as the nurse prayed: "Lord, you were faithful to Abraham, Isaac and Jacob, and we know you care for Mr. Levi. We thank you that you love him and will never forget him. He needs your comfort right now. Please ease his pain and give him strength to bear up under this strain. Amen."

All the muscles in Mr. Levi's body visibly relaxed and the pain subsided following the prayer. Again he held the nurse's hand and wept. Then he went to sleep. From that point on Mr. Levi became more cooperative and less demanding with all the staff. His bladder spasms came less frequently.■

Mr. Levi had grown up with a strong Jewish heritage in which God was remembered for his mighty acts in the history of Israel. But he had also lived through World War 2 in Germany and experienced fear and hopelessness as most of his family and friends died at the hands of other human beings. Auschwitz seemed to have negated any sense of a powerful and loving God for him. Personal suffering had become meaningless and merely contributed to his anger toward God, who he felt had deserted him. His trip to Israel had reminded him of God's faithfulness to his people, even in the midst of suffering and persecution. The nurse's prayer recalled God's care for Abraham, Isaac and Jacob and helped to restore the hope that God had not changed. Mr. Levi could rest in the care of a loving, faithful God who was personally involved with him.

We may never see a patient picketing the nurse's station with a sign reading, "Give me my spiritual rights!" but we may often care for patients like Mr. Levi who are just as obviously waving red flags of pain, fear and anxiety that may reflect an underlying concern for spiritual understanding and support.[5]

The 1973 Code for Nurses adopted by the International Congress of Nursing states that the fourfold responsibility of the nurse is to "promote health, to prevent illness, to restore health and to alleviate suffering. . . .

inherent in nursing is respect for life, dignity and rights of man."[6] A right can be defined as something which is due a person because of a specific claim, moral principle or law, as in the case of the various rights guaranteed people in the United States Constitution.[7] The World Health Organization assumes that spiritual care is a right when it defines health as encompassing the whole person in terms of total fitness for living—as maintaining a state of physical, emotional, spiritual and social well-being, not merely as the absence of disease.

An understanding of the nature of man as a physical, psychosocial and spiritual being is fundamental to both medicine and nursing. Spiritual care is considered to be a right. Yet spiritual needs make no sense at all apart from an understanding of God. The right to receive spiritual understanding ultimately comes from him. Paul expressed this thought in his message to the Athenians. He said that all people were created by God "that they should seek God, in the hope that they might feel after him and find him" (Acts 17:27) in order to establish and maintain a relationship with him that would meet their spiritual needs.

Our understanding of the nurse's role in spiritual care is the result of many influences, including our family background, our nursing education and experience, the institutional policies where we work and the people we work with. Yet none of these factors, alone or in combination, is as strong an influence on us as our own personal system of values that is based on our beliefs about God and man. If we believe that man is created by God and the need for a relationship with God is fundamental to a person's nature, then this need becomes our primary *mandate* to give adequate spiritual care that can promote and help to restore health and contribute to the well-being of the whole person.

I don't think I'm ready to meet God. Can you help me? Does God really care about me, nurse? Why did God let this happen? Who is God and what is man? The way a nurse answers these questions will determine the extent of that nurse's involvement in identifying and meeting a patient's spiritual needs. We cannot give to others what we do not possess ourselves. That does not mean we must have all the answers before we can launch into the spiritual dimension of care with patients. But it does mean we must have a commitment to search for the answers and to know where to go for further help.

Chapter 2
What Is Human?

When I look at thy heavens, the work of thy fingers,
  the moon and the stars which thou hast established;
what is man that thou art mindful of him,
  and the son of man that thou dost care for him?
Psalm 8:3-4

The five senses reveal many things about a person. For example, we can look at Mrs. Jones, a patient just admitted to the emergency room. One look will tell us she is lethargic, dyspneic, overweight and unkempt. We can listen and realize she is disoriented. Her breath smells fruity. Her skin is dry and her pulse is rapid. If we were to test her urine, it would be sweet with glucose. These observations would lead us to suspect diabetic acidosis and to plan care accordingly.

Mrs. Jones may be a diabetic in acidosis, but she is much more than that. The diagnosis we have made through the perception of our senses is not wrong, but it is incomplete. Who is Mrs. Jones? What is she living for? Is she really worth all the time, energy and expense to reverse her acidosis, even though she probably will not take her insulin when she goes home again? Answers to such questions must come from a source outside ourselves. For the purposes of this book that source will be the Bible.

The relationship between God and humanity as portrayed in the Scriptures has two major elements. First, it is a relationship between the Creator and his creature. Second, we are created in God's image (Gen. 1:27). The relationship requires dependency and obedience on our part, but it bestows on us dignity and honor.

God's Creature

We are created *by* God to live in relationship with him. We are also created *for* God (Col. 1:16). God has plans for us whom he created. Therefore, we as creatures are not free to define our own values, goals and limits, but must discover those designed for us by our Creator. God addressed Job as a creature when he said, "Where were you when I laid the foundation of the earth? Tell me, if you have understanding"

(Job 38:4). A basic fact of human existence is that we can never declare ourselves independent from God and still realize our potential.

In the Hebrew mentality, to be alive meant to be in relationship with God. To be out of relationship with God meant death.[1] In fact, the precise time of death was considered to be the moment at which a person ceased to praise God, whether or not he was survived by biological functioning.[2]

The New Testament further expands the concept that a person apart from God is dead (Rom. 6:23). Paul states that when Adam sinned in the Garden of Eden he caused all humankind to be subjected to death (Rom. 5:14; 1 Cor. 15:21). Adam, the creature, refused to stay within the limits set for him by God, the Creator. His disobedience severed the God-man relationship and death ensued.

Why is such a strong term—*death*—applied to those who are out of relationship with God? First of all, a person who is out of relationship with God cuts himself off from the source of love and relationship and becomes self-centered.[3] A self-centered person cannot truly give himself to another person in love and trust. He becomes alienated and fearful. Our society demands that men and women find their worth and identity in themselves and their achievements. Human relationships are valued for what they contribute to that sense of worth and identity. Long-term commitments to others are seen as dull and confining. Competing in a success-oriented world without moral responsibility to or for others is considered "freedom."[4] Such a philosophy may be fulfilling as long as a person remains successful. However, because we are creatures, each of us will eventually fail at something. We come crashing into our own mortality and find we cannot control all the circumstances of our lives. We find we do need other people, and having made that discovery, we also find we need a source of love outside of ourselves. The only dependable source of that love is God.

The second effect of a broken relationship with God is guilt.[5] We have true moral guilt for having severed that relationship, but we also experience another form of guilt. Without a clear understanding of God's view of man, we may set unrealistic goals and standards for ourselves which we cannot fully achieve. Failure to attain our goals makes us feel guilty and deflates our self-image. We may also feel guilty over our inability to be what we want others to think we are. We criticize others to make ourselves look good, then feel guilty about our critical comments, for they have cut us off from those people.[6]

As human beings we find meaning and purpose in the context of relationships.[7] When a person lacks significant relationships, life seems meaningless and purposeless. Human relationships, if not set in the larger context of a relationship with God, easily become exploitative and insecure.[8] Only a relationship with God gives life and relationships true meaning and purpose in the face of failure, suffering and death.[9]

That we are spiritual beings means a relationship with God is basic to our total functioning. From God, we receive love and relate with God through Jesus Christ. Jesus Christ came as the "second Adam" to rescue humanity from death by restoring the God-man relationship. This relationship is described by Jesus as "abundant life" (Jn. 10:10) and "eternal life" (Jn. 3:16). It is the direct opposite of death.

God's Image

Not only are we God's creatures—created by and for God—but we are created in God's "image" (Gen. 1:26). We are made to in some way reflect the character of God and represent him by having "dominion" over creation (Gen. 1:28). Exactly how we reflect God's likeness is not entirely clear and has been a point of conjecture throughout history; but because we are created in the image of God, we can assume that we can come to understand ourselves better as we get to know God. Yet we can never know all there is to know about God, so our own identity remains somewhat of a mystery. Sin, which clouds the image of God in us, further veils our true identity.

The Scriptures assert that God's perfect image is seen in the person of Jesus Christ (Col. 1:15). In Jesus Christ we can come to know both God and ourselves. In his life we see God and humanity in perfect relationship. In his actions we can discern God's purposes for us and realize his compassion for a renegade humanity. In Christ's crucifixion we begin to comprehend the extent of our sin, which required so great a sacrifice, as well as realize the extreme worth God places on humanity which compelled him to make that sacrifice.[10]

Apart from the understanding that we are created in the image of God, human life loses worth and meaning. Vernon Grounds quotes a description of human value which circulated in pre-Hitler Germany: "The human body contains enough fat to make 7 bars of soap, enough iron to make a medium-sized nail, enough phosphorus for 2000 matchheads, and enough sulfur to rid oneself of fleas."[11] Few people would seriously consider measuring human value in such base terms; we do the same thing, however, when we determine a person's value by how much he or she can contribute to society or how much work he or she can produce. The problems of minorities, the handicapped, the elderly and the retarded, and even the hiring and firing practices of industry, demonstrate our society's low view of human worth.

To be created in the image of God makes us thinking, feeling, creative beings. Each person, regardless of our own evaluation of him or her, has worth and honor in the eyes of God. Each person carries the potential to reflect the likeness of his Creator as he enters into a dynamic, personal relationship with God.

An Integrated Whole

As spiritual beings we are naturally psychosocial beings also. To be alive is to strive, to hope, to yearn, to love. A person in relationship thinks, feels, acts and interacts. To *be* is to be a part of—to find identity within a community of significant others where one's uniqueness is appreciated and nurtured. We are complex individuals who need to live in harmony with God, ourselves and other people. We need to sense direction. To establish ultimate meaning and purpose in our lives we need an awareness of being created in God's image. Jesus summed up God's purposes for us by saying, "You shall love the Lord your God with all your heart, and with all your soul, and with all your mind" and "You shall love your neighbor as yourself" (Mt. 22:37, 39). A loving relationship with God overflows into a love for other people and a sense of self-worth.

Spiritual and psychosocial man or woman is also a biological being. The body is extremely important in Judeo-Christian thought. To the writers of the Old Testament, anatomical parts were considered to be the bearers of a person's spiritual and ethical impulses. Physiological functions were believed to created a steady bond with God which maintained life. [12] Psalm 35 provides an example:

All my bones shall say,
  "O LORD, who is like thee,
thou who deliverest the weak
  from him who is too strong for him." (Ps. 35:10)
We feel the effect of a broken relationship with God physically; for
example, Psalm 38:3:
There is no soundness in my flesh
  because of thy indignation;
there is no health in my bones
  because of my sin.
The reverse is also shown to be true. When the physical body is in distress, the entire being, including the person's relationship with God, is
affected. When Job was in the midst of his physical afffliction, he cried
out:
I still rebel and complain against God;
  I cannot keep from groaning.
How I wish I knew where to find him,
  and knew how to go where he is. (Job 23:1-3 TEV)
  The physical body is given special meaning in the Christian faith because Christians believe that God became man in Jesus Christ through
taking on human flesh. The body is the visible expression of the whole
person. Through the body we can enter into relationships. Although the
Scriptures refer to aspects of persons with various terms—translated as
"body," "flesh," "soul," "spirit"—these terms denote dimensions of
wholeness, not parts which can be dissected. For instance, the Hebrew
word *nepes,* which is often translated "soul," could also be translated
"person." In Genesis 2:7 the man became a living *nepes.* A person does
not *possess* a *nepes,* he or she *is* a *nepes.* [13] In the same way we do not
possess a body, we are a body. [14]
  When we look at the English translations of Greek and Hebrew terms
in the Bible, we often interpret them according to a mindset influenced
by Greek philosophy, especially that of Plato. According to Greek philosophy (as well as most Eastern religions), the body is evil and distracting.
The true person is considered to be the spirit, or inner core of the person,
which is inherently good. The evil body imprisons the good spirit. True
spirituality is seen to be the release of the spirit from the body.

This dualistic view leads to a low regard for human life. Adherents to a dualistic philosophy, such as the Gnostics of the first century A.D., demonstrate the moral implications of their view of the body. They go to one of two extremes, either indulging freely in physical pleasures (for example, orgies) or becoming rigidly ascetic (even restraining from sexual relations in marriage). Since only the spirit matters, the body is either scorned or considered irrelevant.[15]

People tend to want ideas put into neat categories and so dualism appears as a tempting option. Human beings, however, cannot be divided into categories. Should dualism form the basis of nursing the implications would be disastrous!

Most nurses intellectually agree that a person is an integrated whole, but they seldom function accordingly. The tendency is to think in terms of two categories: physical needs and psychosocial needs. Some add a third category: spiritual needs. Physical care is usually given top priority. Emotional support is considered important but time-consuming; therefore, it is usually reserved for less hectic moments. Spiritual needs, if considered at all, are generally felt to be the domain of the clergy. Rather than viewing patients as whole persons, nursing practice frequently divides them into prioritized parts.

Case 5. Mrs. Jones (introduced at the beginning of this chapter) was admitted to the hospital. Her acidosis was reversed, her insulin was regulated, and she was discharged with instructions for a 1000 Calorie ADA diet. A week later the public health nurse visited and found her listless and depressed.

She admitted she had not taken her insulin or followed the prescribed diet. As the nurse talked with her, Mrs. Jones began to pour out her feelings of anger, guilt and inability to cope with her alcoholic husband, feelings she had not expressed during her hospitalization. She said she felt like everyone, including God, had abandoned her. "Why should I take care of myself?" she asked the nurse.■

Human beings do have different dimensions, varying ways of expressing themselves, which we perceive as the physical, the psychosocial and the spiritual aspects of being. Illness affects persons in their totality, not merely their bodies or their minds or their spirits. Our nursing care must be focused on the person as a unity. The key to human integration is a relationship with God which permeates the whole being. Through a relationship with God, we find our worth and identity and become free to love and be loved by others. Based on the above understandings our working concept of human beings will be this: *the person is a physically, psychosocially and spiritually integrated being, created to live in harmony with God, himself and others.*

Any statement about the nature of human life is a religious statement. Life draws its definition and finds its meaning and worth from its source. A Christian believes that God is the source of all life; our concept of humanity therefore reflects that belief. Nursing, which grew out of the practical application of the gospel in everyday life, has traditionally held a Christian understanding of humanity. Newer theories, reflecting a growing pluralism in our society, are challenging traditional views.

As innovative models of the nature of human beings are proposed, and as ancient models of Eastern philosophy are revived and imposed in nursing, the nature of nursing will radically change. Many of these models sound impressive and scientific, but if a definition of persons were wholly scientific, we would be back to measuring our worth by the value of the chemicals in our bodies. That is why we want to be clear about our presuppositions from the very beginning. We challenge each nurse to examine the religious and philosophical underpinnings of the concept of humanity under which he or she functions, for what we believe about human life determines how we practice nursing.

Chapter 3
What Are Spiritual Needs?

In our society we have selected the word
"religion" to connote the recognition of Man's
ultimate dependence upon a superior being.
Apart from any denominational position, it
is critical for the nurse to realize that
there is a fundamental view of religion which
simply recognizes a healthy relationship
of man to God, to his fellow man, and to himself
and which is a direct consequence of his
rational spiritual nature. Apart from the influence
of "civilization," man's religious impulses
are spontaneous and fairly uniform. Man has a
marked tendency not only toward dependency
upon but also toward trust in a sovereign
Lord, gratitude toward Him as the great
benefactor, love for Him as the source of endless
goodness and sorrow, and a need for punishment
for having offended Him. These are the
basic concepts of religion with which a nurse can
ill afford non-familiarity.
Sister Mary Hubert

S piritual needs have been a stated concern throughout the history of nursing; however, they have been largely defined either as the frankly religious functions relegated to the clergy or as vague, undefinable entities that cannot be accurately assessed. Baptism, communion, prayer, certain dietary regulations, the keeping of special holy days, regular attendance at a place of worship—these are all legitimate expressions of faith in God and may be important components of a person's normal lifestyle. If illness and hospitalization prevent a person from carrying out any of these practices, one may well feel his or her spiritual needs are not being met.

Yet spiritual needs can be concretely defined in a broader sense. We can move from looking at the symbols, or expressions of a person's relationship with God, to the very essence of that relationship itself. (For a summary of significant research related to assessing spiritual needs of patients, see appendix A.) While it is important for a nurse to respect and recognize the differences in the way a person expresses his or her faith, it is significantly more important that a nurse comprehend how similar are everyone's basic spiritual needs.[1]

We are integrated beings created to live in harmony with God, ourselves and other people. To maintain harmonious relationships, we must first make sure "right" relationships are established. This is similar to composing a piece of music.

A melody is said to be harmonized when other notes that form a chord are sounded at the same time as some of the key notes in the melody. Each note in the chord must be in a certain defined relationship to each of the notes in the melodic line to create a pleasing sound that is rich and full. If these musical laws of composition are not followed, disharmony results.

For man, a harmonious relationship with himself (characterized by a sense of joy and peace) and rich, meaningful relationships with other people can only be truly experienced when a person first establishes and maintains a dynamic and personal relationship with God who is the key to physical, emotional, social and spiritual integration. A lack of relationship with God can lead to discordant relationships, with oneself and with others.

The primary reason for this need for a relationship with God lies in the nature of God, who is both personal and dynamic—actively involved in the world he has created. Paul Steeves describes God the Creator as the holy, almighty God who desires "to enter into direct, intimate, personal relationship with his creatures."[2]

God is also a loving Father. A synonym for relationship which expresses a more intimate connection between God and humans is *kinship*. The apostle Paul, in refuting the idea of an "unknown god" in Athens, quoted a Greek poet as saying, "In him we live and move and have our being. . . . For we are indeed his offspring" (Acts 17:28).

The Bible gives numerous illustrations of what it means to establish and/or maintain a dynamic and personal relationship with God. Perhaps the most notable example is that of a son who decided to leave the home of his father for a far country. The trip proved disastrous. Not only did the son lose all the money he had taken with him, but a great famine arose in the land. This forced him to feed swine to survive. He was very much aware of the absence of meaning and purpose in this sorry state of existence. He also keenly felt a need for love and forgiveness from his father and desired to re-establish a relationship and restore communication. His needs forced him home. Freely offering his love, the father ran and embraced his son before the son arrived at the gate. The son then confessed his sin of disobedience and was rewarded by an even greater outpouring of the father's love as a huge banquet was prepared in his honor. He was now able to receive the full benefits of sonship.[3]

God is a father to all people in the sense of giving all people life and breath. But the Fatherhood of God and the resulting benefits of sonship can only be fully realized when a person is able to experience God as the source of meaning and purpose, love and relatedness, and forgiveness. These are three factors which contribute to the establishment and maintenance of a dynamic and personal relationship with God.

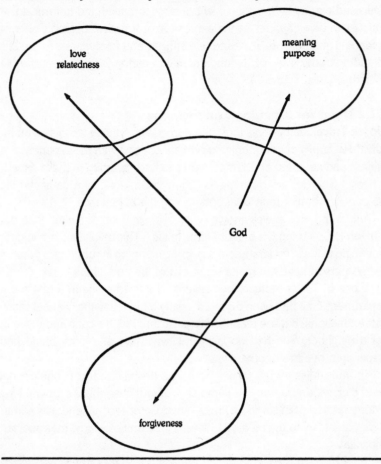

Figure 1. God as the Source

A lack of any one of these three factors will produce a spiritual need, which can be simply defined: *A spiritual need is the lack of any factor or factors necessary to establish and/or maintain a dynamic, personal relationship with God.*[4]

Because God is the source of these factors, a relationship is established and maintained as an individual responds to God in obedience, according to the grace God has offered. Illness and other forms of crisis can impair a person's ability to sense God's desire for a relationship and can make a person feel hopeless, unloved and unforgiven. A nurse can be a channel for the expression to a patient of God's offer of meaning and purpose, love and relatedness, and forgiveness. An understanding of these factors is fundamental to caring for patients as whole persons. (See Figure 2.)

The Need for Meaning and Purpose

Joyce Travelbee believes that "the purpose of nursing is to assist an individual, family or community to prevent or cope with the experience of illness and suffering and, if necessary, to find meaning in these experiences." She defines meaning as "the reason given to a particular life experience by the individual undergoing the experience."[5]

Viktor Frankl, a well-known Viennese psychiatrist, writes that our search for meaning is a primary force in life.[6] This involves searching for meaning to life in general and discovering meaning in suffering in particular. A person needs to make sense out of life and illness.

Case 6. Miss Morgan, age seventy-six, lived alone in a one-room apartment. She had been declared legally blind following bilateral cataract extractions, but she managed to get around with a cane and the help of a neighbor. She had no living relatives. Her one close friend had recently moved to another state.

In June Miss Morgan's neighbor was hospitalized with pneumonia and died within two weeks. Three days after the neighbor's funeral Miss Morgan attempted suicide with an overdose of seconal and was admitted, comatose, to the medical intensive care unit of a large metropolitan hospital.

Miss Morgan recovered within four days and was transferred to the psychiatric wing. After a week of therapy she was visited by her medical doctor who informed her rather abruptly that she would be moved to a nursing home "as soon as there was an available bed." Miss Morgan burst into tears. A nurse passing the room overheard the conversation and stopped in after the doctor left. "How are you feeling?" the nurse asked.

"Like an aborted baby! I'm a nobody!" Miss Morgan exclaimed. "Nobody loves me, needs me or wants me. There's no meaning in life—no

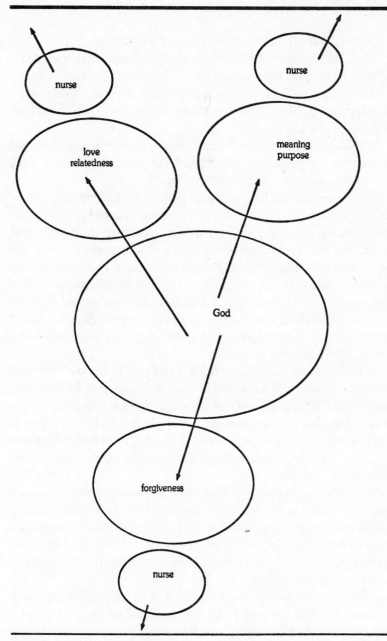

Figure 2. A Nurse as the Channel

purpose for living. I want to leave this nice world."

"Has God been of any help to you in all of this?" asked the nurse, touching Miss Morgan on the shoulder.

Miss Morgan pulled away and rolled toward the wall. "God! God!" she cried angrily. "What God? I don't want to talk about God. There is no God. Can't you see that?"■

The German philosopher Friedrich Nietzsche summed up the need for meaning and purpose in suffering with the statement, "He who has a *why* to live can bear with almost any *how.*"[7]

Miss Morgan did not have a *why*. In the past, life had meaning in relationship to other people. Meaning had also been related to her own self-sufficiency—a successful career, an alert, intelligent mind and good health. She could no longer see or walk and was unable to make any decisions about her future. Miss Morgan saw life as a laborious task to be performed. She preferred death (which she later described as a "state of nothingness") to an empty and purposeless existence, devoid of significant human relationships. Her perceptions of a world that was cold and uncaring and of a God who was nonexistent produced feelings of alienation and worthlessness.

Life *is* a task, concurs Frankl. But the way people approach that task may differ and affect their ability to cope with crisis and find meaning and purpose in the experience of suffering. Frankl believes that the difference between the religious and the apparently irreligious person is that the religious person experiences his existence not merely as a task but as a mission, and is aware of his taskmaster, the source of his mission. That source is God.[8]

In the Bible we have a graphic example of a man who was very much aware of his taskmaster. The man's name was Job.[9] He was considered deeply religious. He worshiped God and was faithful to keep the religious customs of the day. Yet despite Job's awareness of God in his life, when confronted with personal tragedy he was unable to see meaning and purpose in the experience.

Job's crisis was brought on by the death of his ten children, the death of his servants, sheep and cattle, and tremendous personal physical distress in the form of boils that covered his entire body. Job also lost the respect of his family and friends. He continually asked the question,

"Why me?" He welcomed death. At one point Job cried out to the Lord in despair:

Human life is like forced army service,
  like a life of hard manual labor,
  like a slave longing for cool shade;
  like a worker waiting for his pay.
Month after month I have nothing to live for;
  night after night brings me grief. . . .
My days pass by without hope,
  pass faster than a weaver's shuttle . . .
I give up; I am tired of living.
Leave me alone. My life makes no sense. (Job 7:1-3, 6, 16 TEV)

Job's tragic story continued until one day God spoke to Job directly and gave him hope.

The reader of Job's story has the benefit of knowing that the underlying cause of his suffering was a direct attack of Satan to test Job's faithfulness to God. God did not reveal this *why* to Job as the reason for his suffering. Instead, God told Job that it was enough to know that God himself was in complete control of Job's suffering even as he was in control of the entire universe. This fact brought security without the need for more specific answers. William Hulme says the reason for this security was that Job now knew the *who* in a new way. The *who* was God himself.[10] Job's knowledge of God was increased. His relationship with God was deepened. This caused Job to confess,

I know, LORD, that you are all-powerful;
  that you can do everything you want.
You ask how I dare question your wisdom
  when I am so very ignorant.
I talked about things I did not understand,
  about marvels too great for me to know.
You told me to listen while you spoke
  and to try to answer your questions.
Then I knew only what others had told me,
  but now I have seen you with my own eyes.
So I am ashamed of all I have said
  and repent in dust and ashes. (Job 42:1-6 TEV)

This admission brought Job beyond the summary of meaning given by Nietzsche to a greater degree of understanding. It is not he who knows the *why* but he who knows the *Who* that can bear with any suffering. Hulme says this leaves room for faith and makes pressing questions less pressing.[11] The fact that God is in control gives meaning and purpose to any situation.

Some degree of hope is possible without a knowledge of God's control yet this hope is basically insecure. Placing ultimate hope for deliverance from a crisis situation in ourselves, in other people or in the possibility of changing circumstances may be mere wishful thinking. People are often disappointed.

Hoping in God may not mean an abrupt end to a crisis. Hope in God is not dependent on God's ability to deliver a person from difficult circumstances (though God certainly can and frequently does) but on God's control of the circumstances and his ability to support a person in the midst of them. This can lead to a deeper relationship with God, to emotional and spiritual growth, and to the ability to help other people in their crises. The apostle Paul relates an account of hoping in God in the middle of a crisis that was threatening to crush him. He was comforted by God in the midst of this, was later delivered and then able to comfort a large company of people who were facing similar adverse circumstances (2 Cor. 1:3-11).

Hope has been defined as "a glimmer of something better."[12] Meaning and purpose for life and meaning and purpose in suffering can be found in a person's relationship with God and the knowledge of his control.

But even this present relationship and knowledge could not provide hope forever without the possibility of a meaningful and purposeful future. That hope ultimately depends on the promise of eternal fellowship with God which continues on after this present life on earth ends. The Bible equates hope and deliverance in the Old Testament with the coming Messiah,[13] and in the New Testament with the arrival of that Messiah, Jesus.[14] Jesus enables a person to have an eternal relationship with God. Ultimate meaning and purpose lie in the possibility of this long-term relationship and God's promise to end all suffering and restore harmonious relationships—man with God, himself and others—for those who hope in him through his Son, Jesus.[15]

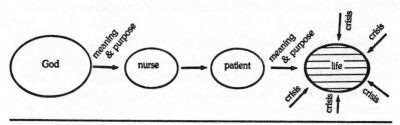

Figure 3. Meaning and Purpose

A person who senses God's direction in his life is able to adapt to unexpected changes. He has hope even when his usual support systems fail him. He knows that God will never fail him. A nurse can assist a patient in finding meaning and purpose in life and in crisis by being a catalyst in his relationship with God.

The Need for Love and Relatedness

"During the nineteenth century," writes anthropologist Ashley Montagu, "more than half the infants in their first year of life regularly died from a disease called *marasmus,* a Greek word meaning 'wasting away.'" This disease, which was also known as infantile atrophy or debility, was characterized by a gradual loss of flesh and strength for no apparent reason. Montagu goes on to say that as late as the second decade of the twentieth century the death rate for infants under one year of age in various foundling institutions of the United States was nearly one hundred per cent. The cause of marasmus was not identified until after World War 2 when specific studies were undertaken. The cause was found to be a lack of mothering. A child, to prosper both physically and emotionally, needs to be carried, caressed, cuddled, and cooed to, in short, a child needs to be loved.[16]

A need for love and relatedness is fulfilled in the context of significant human relationships. Though ways of expressing love may vary, the need does not cease to exist when a child becomes an adult. It may, in fact, intensify. In adulthood the loss of a human relationship that has been the primary source of love and support can contribute to depression or even cause a desire for death. The case study of Miss Morgan illustrates this. A need for love and relatedness goes hand in hand with a need for meaning and purpose.

Masumi Toyotome writes that the security and satisfaction of being loved by someone is basic to a happy life. There are at least three kinds of love, he says, that can determine a person's happiness or lack of happiness: the *if* kind of love, the *because of* kind of love and the *in spite of* kind of love.[17]

The *if* kind of love can be summed up in the sentence, "*If* you satisfy my needs, *then* I will love you." It is a love with strings attached, a conditional love motivated by self-interest. Unfortunately, the *if* kind of love is very common. It causes marriages to break up and can lead to suicide if a person feels he just does not measure up to the standards set for him by others. Nurses will frequently care for patients whose experience of love has been with the *if* variety. Mr. Doe may be in excruciating pain but be afraid that if he cries out the nurse who is caring for him will become annoyed and reject him. Mr. Doe's perceptions may reflect a history of having to measure up to the expectations of others.

The *because of* kind of love is also common and can be reflected in these statements: "I love you because of who you are." "I love you because of what you have." "I love you because of what you do." The burden of having to earn the love of another person may be absent, but another, even greater, burden of fear be present. "What if I lose the very thing I am being loved *because of?*" A young mother facing a hysterectomy may confide to the nurse, "I'm afraid my husband won't love me after my operation because I won't be able to bear him any more children." A man with paraplegia may feel the burden of not measuring up to his wife's expectations of the ideal husband. Any form of illness can reinforce a belief that the ill person has never really been loved for themselves alone.

The *in spite of* kind of love is vastly different and far superior to the other two. Says Toyotome, "One may be the most ugly, most wretched, most debased person in the world and would still be loved when he meets this 'in spite of' kind of love. He does not have to deserve it. He does not have to earn it by being good or attractive or wealthy. He is simply loved as he is, in spite of the faults or ignorance or bad habits or evil records he may have. He may seem absolutely worthless, and yet he would be loved as though he were of infinite worth. This is the kind of love for which our hearts are desperately hungry."[18] An older lady faced with the prospect of a nursing home or a young mother facing a hysterectomy, a paraplegic or a person with a colostomy, severe burns or some other disfigurement could be in special need of the *in spite of* kind of love and relationships which reflect it. This is the kind of love God offers a person.

The *in spite of* kind of love has no strings attached. It is a love that makes no demands other than that the person be open to receive it. God takes the initiative to reach out and love people, but he does not force love on a person. A recognition of this offer of love from God can help draw a person into a meaningful relationship with God and can sustain a relationship that may be a bit shaky as a result of the experience of illness.

Self-pity, depression, insecurity, isolation, desperation and fear are some of the indications of a need for love from oneself, other people and God. Feelings of self-worth, joy, security, belonging, hope and courage are experienced on the other end of the spectrum when the need for love is met.[19] These are the benefits of the *in spite of* kind of love God offers to people when they are going through a crisis.

"There is no fear in love," states the First Epistle of John, "but perfect love casts out fear" (4:18). Fear has been defined as "the painful emotion that arises at the thought that we may be harmed or made to suffer [and] persists while we are subject to the will of someone who does not desire our well-being. The moment we come under the protection of one of good will, fear is cast out."[20]

Illness can intensify fear. In the first chapter of this book we met Mr. Levi, who was in pain and very fearful. He was reminded of God's love for him as he reflected on God's faithfulness to his people in the past. A knowledge of God's presence seems to be one key to experiencing his love. This goes beyond the fact of God's being in control of the situation. While the fact of God's control can be a comfort in itself, the kind of God who is in control is equally important to a sufferer who needs to know a God who desires his best good.

Isaiah 43 expresses this aspect of God's character. It pictures a loving God who promises to walk with a person through crisis:

When you pass through the waters I will be with you;
  and through the rivers, they shall not overwhelm you;
when you walk through the fire you shall not be burned,
  and the flame shall not consume you.
For I am the LORD your God,
  the Holy One of Israel, your Savior. (Is. 43:2-3)

This passage continues with a reminder to the Israelites that they are precious in God's eyes, that they are honored and that he loves them. "Fear not," says God, "for I am with you" (Is. 43:5).

A person experiences the love of God when he or she is able to hope in God. The writer of Psalm 42 uses his memory of the past to give him hope in the present. This enables him to recall God's faithfulness and steadfast love:

Why are you cast down, O my soul,
  and why are you disquieted within me?
Hope in God; for I shall again praise him,
  my help and my God.
My soul is cast down within me,
  therefore I remember thee
from the land of Jordan and of Hermon,
  from Mount Mizar. . . .
By day the LORD commands his steadfast love;
  and at night his song is with me,
  a prayer to the God of my life. (Ps. 42:5-6, 8)

God as Creator is in control of every situation. God as Father cares about the people who are suffering. A loving parent who wants his child to grow up to be able to function responsibly in the world does not shield his child from all painful experiences. The parent does provide support and encouragement as the child struggles through the frustrations of life. God, as a loving, concerned Father, does not protect his children from all suffering, but he does promise to go with them through it. The spiritual and emotional growth which can occur as a result of suffering may not be immediately observable or necessarily welcomed, but it can be a source of hope and courage.

A person who is experiencing God's love is able to see himself as a person of worth. This frees him to love God, himself and other people. A

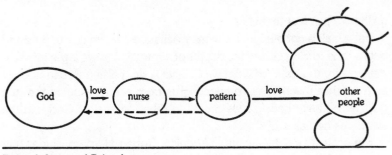

Figure 4. Love and Relatedness

nurse becomes a channel of God's love to a patient when the nurse communicates God's *in spite of* kind of love and faithful presence in crisis. The nurse may restore hope by helping the patient remember God's presence with him in the past and helping him realize that God is also with him in his present illness.

The Need for Forgiveness

In the first chapter of his book *Whatever Became of Sin?* psychiatrist Karl Menninger describes a scene that took place in Chicago in September 1972. A plainly dressed man, standing on a busy street corner, was repeating over and over again one word—*Guilty!* Each time the man said the word he would point to a passing pedestrian. The response, says Menninger, was extraordinary, almost eerie. The people's behavior indicated that they actually *felt* guilty.[21]

Guilt is waiting to point a finger at us on *every* corner. Paul Tournier, a Swiss physician, concludes that "a guilty conscience is the seasoning of our daily life."[22]

We may first experience guilt as a child when our behavior does not measure up to the standards set for us by our parents. We disobey them and do the very things we are told not to do. Guilt rears its ugly head again at the other end of life in the form of regrets not only for the things we have done but for the many things we have failed to accomplish.

Guilt often results from the failure to live up to one's own expectations or the expectations of others. This failure may not relate as much to our own inabilities as to unrealistic expectations imposed on us which are impossible to meet. This can create false guilt. We are not really guilty; we just feel that way.

False guilt is not benign. It can incapacitate us, eating up our time and energy and forcing us into the depths of depression as we lapse into self-pity and try to atone for what we believe is sin. False guilt can also act as a defense mechanism, preventing us from acknowledging the true guilt we all have because we are all in rebellion against God and the standards he has set.[23]

Sin against God makes us truly guilty. Robert Horn concludes that true sin "does not merely bring guilt-feelings, but actually incurs guilt, which shuts us out of God's presence, whether we feel the force of that or not. Sooner or later it also brings guilt-feelings: the sense of shame, the knowledge that we cannot look God in the eye, the fear of Him turning His searching gaze on us."[24]

A group of nurses were asked to describe guilt feelings they had experienced at one time or another. The list was lengthy and included feelings of paranoia, hostility, worthlessness and defensiveness. Behaviors and attitudes were also identified that affected their relationships with others: "I cry and withdraw and have various psychosomatic complaints." "I rationalize a lot, trying to convince myself the guilt isn't really there." "I'm critical of myself, others and God." "I look for a scapegoat." They were also asked to describe their feelings following confession of sin. They admitted to feelings of joy, peace and elation: "I felt cleansed, free." "I had a renewed sense of self-worth." "I was very much aware of restored fellowship with God."[25]

Confession of sin is the means God has given human beings to pave the way to receive forgiveness. One expression of true guilt and a recognition of God's solution is found in Psalm 51.

Have mercy on me, O God,
according to thy steadfast love;
according to thy abundant mercy blot out my transgressions.
Wash me thoroughly from my iniquity,
and cleanse me from my sin!
For I know my transgressions,
and my sin is ever before me.
Against thee, thee only, have I sinned,
and done that which is evil in thy sight,

so that thou art justified in thy sentence
  and blameless in thy judgment. . . .
Purge me with hyssop, and I shall be clean;
  wash me, and I shall be whiter than snow.
Fill me with joy and gladness;
  let the bones which thou hast broken rejoice. (Ps. 51:1-4, 7-8)

We see another example of the need for forgiveness from God in Psalm 32 and the close relationship of unconfessed sin to physical infirmities and mental and emotional symptoms. The psalmist is apparently writing after-the-fact; having experienced God's forgiveness, he reflects back on what has happened to him:

Blessed is he whose transgression is forgiven,
  whose sin is covered. . . .
When I declared not my sin, my body wasted away
  through my groaning all day long.
For day and night thy hand was heavy upon me;
  my strength was dried up as by the heat of summer.
I acknowledged my sin to thee,
  and I did not hide my iniquity;
I said, "I will confess my transgressions to the LORD";
  then thou didst forgive the guilt of my sin. (Ps. 32:1, 3-5)

Peter Ford, in *The Healing Trinity*, gives a striking modern-day example of the adverse effects of unconfessed sin.

Case 7.   The wife of a Protestant minister committed adultery with a member of her husband's congregation. Her inability to confess her infidelity to her husband resulted in manifold physical symptoms including weight loss, abdominal cramping, frequent liquid stools and insomnia. Dr. Ford encouraged confession. She was finally able to do this, her husband forgave her, and her health immediately began to improve. But three months later the symptoms returned with increased depression, vomiting and intractable headaches. The cause? Her inability to accept God's forgiveness and to forgive and accept herself. When she was finally able to do both, she became restored to complete health.[26]■

G. Keith Parker, in a study of patients with kidney disease, says that "guilt is the most important psychological and religious stress related to chronic illness [and] is affected by the patient's ability to cope with it both in psychological and religious terms." He describes an example of this:

Case 8. One patient was so burdened with guilt that it adversely affected not only his relationships with others but also his dialysis treatment. His first wife had died some years earlier on their honeymoon due to his negligent driving. He saw his kidney disease as a punishment from God. When asked what he thought was the greatest sin he replied, "Murder, harder to be forgiven for that than anything else."

He was constantly trying to placate God but could never believe that God could really forgive him and never became free of what Parker calls the "albatross of guilt."[27]

Guilt is a complex problem as the previous case studies illustrate. It can never be dealt with effectively by rationalizing, denying its existence or promising to do better the next time. A true and lasting solution to the problem of guilt can only come when a person confesses his sin, admits his own inability to rid himself of it and exercises faith. Faith might be simply defined as *putting our trust in someone else to do what we cannot do for ourselves.*

Horn compares a person in need of God's forgiveness to a drowning man, flailing his arms around in a futile attempt to rescue himself. Only when he stops trying to save himself, admits defeat and reaches out to his friend who has jumped into the water to help him can he expect to be rescued. He must have faith in his rescuer. He must trust him completely.[28]

The Bible describes God as faithful and trustworthy. He both desires and is able to forgive man and rescue him from the sin of rebellion that results in spiritual death. God's desire to forgive is related to his love which was manifested in the person of Jesus Christ. Jesus came into the world to forgive human beings and to enable us to establish and maintain harmonious relationships with God. He made forgiveness possible by his death on the cross by becoming our substitute, *taking* upon himself our sin and *giving* himself as a sin offering to God.[29]

Yet this forgiveness is not automatically conferred on all people. It is given to those who are willing to receive it. To receive forgiveness a person must confess his rebellion, admit his own helplessness and place his trust in Jesus as the only one who is able to save him and restore him to a dynamic, personal relationship with God.[30]

A person becomes a Christian when a relationship with God is established through faith in Jesus Christ. He is adopted into God's family.[31] This new Father-son relationship that has been established has many benefits, chief of which are peace with God and the promise of eternal life with God after death.[32]

When a person establishes a relationship with God, he or she does not automatically stop sinning. But he does develop new attitudes, desires and behaviors that are a result of the Holy Spirit working in his life to help him grow in his relationship to God, himself and other people. He will have a greater awareness of sin and be more sensitive to his need for forgiveness when he disobeys God in the future. A harmonious relationship with God can be *maintained* when a person confesses subsequent sin and trusts Christ to forgive and to cleanse him.[33]

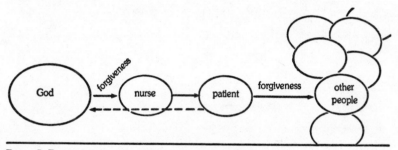

Figure 5. Forgiveness

A person who knows God's forgiveness can be at peace with God, himself and other people. He has a new awareness of God as his Father who gives life meaning and purpose. He can also experience God's love which will in turn enable him to love God, himself and others.

Guilt *is* a complex problem. It may often require the intervention of someone skilled in counseling such as a pastor or a hospital chaplain. A nurse should refer appropriately. A nurse can also become a channel for communicating God's forgiveness as the nurse points a patient to Jesus Christ—the source of forgiveness.

Chapter·4
Spiritual Needs and the Nursing Process

I Wish I Knew You, Mrs. Toby

Lord, you know Mrs. Toby in room 528—
I wish I knew her like you do.

Just now I tiptoed into her darkened room.
She was sleeping soundly—curled up in the
   fetal position she always maintains.
"Mrs. Toby...Mrs. Toby." It was hard to wake her.
"I have your medicine...." No response.
I placed some of the applesauce and crushed
   pills on the end of a tongue blade and
   gently touched it to her lips.
She opened and swallowed—opened and swallowed...
like a baby bird being fed by it's mother.

But Lord! She isn't a baby bird!!
Who is she? What is she really like?
Was she a gourmet cook once upon a time?
Did she like barbecues and Sunday school picnics?

I look at the bed linen and see small blotches of dried blood.
Ugly decubiti cover her shoulders, hips and heels.
Her skin is red, rough and dry.
Bandages and sheepskin pads try to hide ugly wounds,
but they are unsuccessful,

What was she once like, Lord?
Was she a lily of the valley, or did she turn
    tawny in summer?
Was she once soft and smooth like velvet?

We turn Mrs. Toby onto her side.
She moans and cries softly.
Is it the contractures or the decubiti that cause her pain?
I wish you could talk, Mrs. Toby. . . .
I wish you could tell me where you hurt.

What were you like growing up, Mrs. Toby?
Were you the Belle of the Ball or did you hate balls?
Did you prefer climbing trees and fishing for trout?
Were you gentle as a summer breeze
or did you crackle as lightning?
Did you run track, or read poetry by Sara Teasdale?
Lord—I see this twisted body with my eyes.
But Lord—I need your eyes to see the real Mrs. Toby.
Lord—please give me your eyes,
so I can know Mrs. Toby.

Geri Rush Harms, R.N.

Although spiritual needs are recognized as important by many nursing educators,[1] spiritual care is often avoided in the actual delivery of patient care. What prevents us from assessing and meeting spiritual needs?

The major objection of most nurses to meeting the spiritual needs of patients is the feeling that a patient's relationship with God is a private matter into which we should not pry. Yet we inquire without hesitation about bowel movements and menstrual periods. Nursing is an intimate profession. We move into areas of functioning which patients would perform personally and privately if they were able. Spiritual intervention is appropriate if we care about our patients' spiritual life as much as we care about their physical and emotional well-being.

How many times have you been in a social situation in which someone has said to you, "You're a nurse; let me tell you about my operation"? The person begins to pour out all sorts of information and feelings. You feel embarrassed, hearing it in that context. People expect nurses to be interested and to care about their innermost secrets. The public image of the nurse (and hopefully we will never lose it entirely) is of an "angel of mercy." We do not always like being seen according to someone else's image of what we ought to be, but the role often works to our advantage. If we are perceived as concerned, caring people, we frequently have a short cut to rapport and intimacy.

Our relationships with patients are often short term—limited by the amount of time a patient requires nursing care. Except in rare instances, our involvement is only during the course of the illness. While these factors pose some difficulties for us, they may also be advantages. We encounter a patient in weakness. We have never known him or her as a strong, self-sufficient person, so he does not usually feel he has to maintain an image of strength. When illness affects a person's faith, he may feel more comfortable talking about it to a nurse than with others who are close to him. Too often well-meaning people will respond to a strong person who begins to doubt God with comments like, "Don't talk like that. Of course God cares about you!" An unbeliever who suddenly realizes his need for God may feel even more humiliated when he hears, or expects to hear, "What's with this God-talk, George? You never seemed too interested in God before." A nurse comes with no preconceived ideas or expectations about a patient's relationship with God, which makes it less threatening for him to express his doubts and fears—provided we are open to listening.

While we relate to a patient in the context of his illness, we relate to the person not the illness. The hospital is our home turf. We are comfortable there. Most people in a patient's world, his family and friends, may be focusing on the illness more than on the person who is ill. They will not know what to say as they attempt to handle their feelings. They have known the patient when he was healthy and active. The illness poses a personal threat when it strikes a loved one. It changes the nature of the relationships. It is a solemn reminder that "it could happen to me." Awkward barriers are created which prevent free communication of support and concern.

A nurse may be one of the few people who can stand with a patient in his suffering and help him deal with it. Illness is a confrontation with mortality and with ultimate values. A person's relationship with God is part of that confrontation. We must stand ready to assist the patient in his personal struggle.

Crisis is an unscheduled event. When a patient needs help, frequently a nurse is the only one available. An event of the day, or the long, dark, fear-filled hours of the night may bring on a spiritual crisis.

Case 9. Mrs. Sullivan was a seventy-year-old woman with severe burns of the chest, arms and hands. Every evening she would ask for a priest. Each time, the nurse would try unsuccessfully to get a priest to come. Her condition was not critical, so she rated low priority on their schedule of calls. Finally the nurse asked about giving assistance. Mrs. Sullivan said, "Well, I don't think so. I feel guilty that I haven't been to

Mass. I'd like communion. There's something else, too. . . . I can't sleep because every time I close my eyes I see fire and I get afraid. I was hoping the priest would say a prayer for me." The nurse offered to pray for her. Mrs. Sullivan looked skeptical, but agreed. The nurse prayed and Mrs. Sullivan relaxed. The priest came at a later time and brought her communion. ■

Nursing personnel are the only persons available to a patient at the push of a button. We may be rushed and distracted, but we are there.

In many ways nurses represent the health-care community to a patient. Spiritual intervention can give a patient a sense of security and comfort in what may be a frightening, sterile, foreign environment. Prayer, the Scriptures and conversation about spiritual things can provide a link with the familiar and a reminder of God's faithfulness in the past. They can also create a sense of unity and cooperation between a patient and a nurse. If the patient is confident that the nurse is in touch with God, a feeling of trust may develop. In many cases that trust will be extended to the entire hospital community.

A nurse who offers spiritual consolation and encouragement is not usurping the position of the clergy. Travelbee states, "A nurse does not strive only to alleviate physical pain or render physical care—she ministers to the person. The nurse cares for the individual, not a body part. The existence of suffering, whether physical, mental or spiritual *is* the proper concern of the nurse."[2]

We have a responsibility, as nurses, to care for the whole person, including his spiritual needs. A Christian nurse also has a responsibility to integrate faith and nursing practice by offering spiritual consolation and encouragement. Luther spoke of this as the "priesthood of all believers." God calls each of us to minister to others in our own situations.[3] Meeting spiritual needs of patients is one way the nurse exercises this priesthood.

To minister responsibly as a nurse, we must intervene in the context of the nursing process. (See Figure 6.) The nursing process is an ongoing cycle of observing, interpreting, planning, implementing and evaluating (reobserving and reinterpreting). Perhaps more than in any other dimension of human need, spiritual needs are discerned through the interpretation of observations and the testing of hypotheses. Seldom is there a clear set of signs and symptoms of a spiritual need. Two nurses may

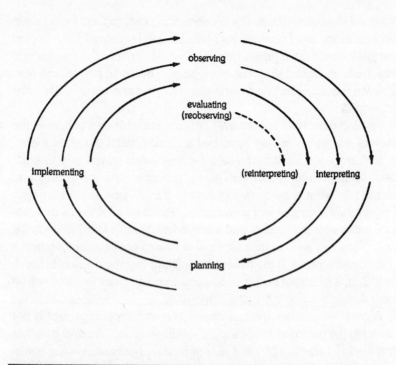

Figure 6. The Nursing Process

care for the same patient, and one of them will discover glaring spiritual needs while the other will find no spiritual needs at all. Assessing spiritual needs requires a sensitive ear and a willingness to respond to tiny clues.

A person's thoughts and feelings about God may well be very personal and precious. To risk having those beliefs challenged or ignored, at a time when a person's world is already shattered by crisis, is difficult. If a nurse responds with warmth and encouragement when a patient speaks tentatively about God, faith, prayer or other spiritual concerns, further verbalization may be forthcoming. Other clues about spiritual needs will be found in a patient's attitudes, behavior, interpersonal relationships and environment. An alert nurse recognizes that beyond surface appearances there may well be deeper meanings.

Assessing spiritual needs is not as difficult or mysterious as it might appear. Often, however, we construct our own barriers to assessment. A patient may express his or her spiritual needs clearly, but these may go undetected because we are hesitant to consider them. We often practice "programmed listening" and filter out what we do not want to hear. If we feel competent in one area but incompetent in another, we may only hear what we feel we can handle confidently. For example:

Pt: I have this terrible cough. I keep praying it will go away. I'm afraid of what it might mean.

Ns: I'll get you some cough medicine.

Or

Pt: Why does God allow me to suffer so?

Ns: I have your pain shot. You'll feel better in a few minutes.

These examples seem obvious on paper, but in actual situations such interactions are more common than we would like to admit. We respond at our level of confidence. But if we have a commitment to caring for the whole person, we cannot claim lack of competence, lack of interest or lack of responsibility in the area of spiritual needs. The assessment of spiritual needs and the appropriate intervention are essential ingredients of the nursing process.

Observing

The first step in the nursing process is to observe the patient. What kinds of things can a nurse observe which might indicate the presence of a spiritual need?

Affect and attitude. Does the patient appear lonely, depressed, angry, anxious or agitated?

Behavior. Does the patient appear to pray before meals or at other times? Does he or she read religious literature? Does he complain frequently, need unusually high doses of sedation or pace the halls at night? Does he joke inappropriately?

Verbalization. Does the patient mention God, prayer, faith, church or religious topics (even briefly)? Does he ask about a visit from the clergy? Does he express fear of death?

Interpersonal relationships. Who visits? How does the patient respond to visitors? Does his or her minister come? How does the patient relate with other patients and nursing personnel? Is he a loner?

Environment. Does the patient have a Bible, prayer book, devotional literature, religious medals or a rosary in his room? Are his or her get-well cards religious? Does his church send him altar flowers or Sunday bulletins?

Interpreting

Observations alone cannot form the basis for nursing care. The next step in the nursing process is to determine the meaning of the clues observed. It is at this stage that a nurse may indicate to a patient an openness to discuss spiritual matters by communicating a concern about his or her thoughts and feelings, and a willingness to stand with him or her through struggles.

Assumptions cannot be made about a patient's affect and attitude. Observations must be tested. By reflecting a patient's mood, a nurse may enable a patient to verbalize his or her feelings. For example, the nurse might say, "You seem sad today, Mr. Gray." It is important to keep the reflections open-ended. The temptation for a nurse is to tack on questions such as, "What can I do to make you feel better?" This shifts the focus away from the patient and his feelings and onto the nurse. If a patient is allowed to verbalize feelings, a bond of trust will usually be established with a nurse who takes the time to listen. Frequently, feelings expressed will stem from needs for meaning, love or forgiveness.

A person's behavior can be an important clue to his or her beliefs, but it can also be misleading. For instance, a patient's wife, who waited anxiously outside of the intensive care unit clutching a rosary, appeared to be a Roman Catholic who was praying. She turned out to be Jewish, and she carried an assortment of other objects she considered good luck charms. In another instance, a patient in the coronary care unit was ordered on strict bedrest. He was found on the floor by his bed several evenings in a row. Finally, a nurse asked him why he kept getting out of bed and discovered it was his usual custom to pray kneeling beside his bed each night before going to sleep. Behavior is often a manifestation of spiritual distress. A conscientious nurse will probe beneath the surface to discover an action's meaning.

Interpersonal relationships can be significant indicators of a patient's spiritual well-being or distress. What do the patients' visits and visitors mean to him or her? Does a lack of visitors indicate a lack of meaningful relationships? Has the patient notified anyone that he is in the hospital? Does his family have transportation problems? Are there other problems at home? Does a large number of visitors mean a strong support system or many superficial acquaintances? Can the patient be honest with his friends and family, or does he feel he must maintain a façade? Does his pastor visit? Do other members of his church or religious group visit? Does he appreciate these visits?

Observing a patient's affect and behavior after visitors leave, and validating those observations, can be helpful in interpreting how the person feels about his relationships.

Case 10. Mr. Wright seemed angry and became uncooperative after his pastor visited. The nurse reflected the change in his behavior to him. He replied, "Do you know what the pastor told me? He said he knew I wasn't right with God because he had seen me smoking . . . **because of** that he said I'd go to hell if I die while I'm in the hospital."

Mr. Wright's family had rallied behind the pastor, hoping that his scare tactics would make Mr. Wright stop smoking as the doctor had ordered. Instead, this left him feeling totally isolated, angry and cut off from his pastor, his family and God. ■

A patient's behavior toward personnel can be a strong indicator of his relationships with significant others. If a person is uncooperative, aggressive, demanding or withdrawn for no apparent reason, the behavior may stem from difficulties in significant relationships, including a person's relationship with God.

Articles in a patient's room may reflect his or her concerns, values and beliefs. Photographs often indicate significant relationships. Gifts and cards may give further insight into the patient's relationships. Are they religious, humorous, personal? Bibles, devotional books, religious objects and cards in the room may reflect the patient's concerns or the concerns of his friends or relatives. A nurse can tactfully comment on these environmental clues in such a way that the patient can respond at a feeling level. For example, "I see you have a Bible here. Do you have a favorite Bible passage?" That question can be followed by, "What do you especially like about that passage?" Often the patient's response will indicate his concerns at the moment as well as give clues about his religious background. For instance, a person may reply, "The twenty-third psalm is my favorite because I memorized it as a child, and it reminds me that God is with me, even now."

An evaluation of the strength and meaning of a patient's religious practices can prove valuable in assisting him to establish and/or maintain a dynamic, personal relationship with God. A nurse may then intervene more specifically at the patient's level of faith and understanding. The questions in Table 1 can be useful in gathering data in order to enter the patient's religious world as a helping person.

Table 1. Religious Values Clarification[4]

Goal A: To understand a person's beliefs about and involvement with God and religious practice.
1. Are there any religious practices which are important to you? If so, could you tell me about them?
2. How is God involved in your life?
3. How would you describe God?

Goal B: To determine the extent to which a person's religious practices serve as a resource for faith and life.
1. Do you feel your faith is helpful to you? How is it helpful?
2. Is prayer important to you? In what ways?
3. Is the Bible, or any other religious book, helpful to you? How?
4. Have any events or experiences changed your feelings about God? Has your present illness made any difference in your faith?

Goal C: To assess whether a person's resources for hope and strength are founded on reality.
1. In what ways is your faith important to you right now?
2. What helps you most when you feel afraid or alone?
3. Is there anything you are hoping for right now?
4. What is your source of strength right now?

Goal D: To give a person an opportunity to accept spiritual help.
1. How can I help you in carrying out your faith?
2. Would you like me to pray for you? read the Bible to you? (and so on, according to cues given by the patient).
3. Would you like a visit from your pastor or the hospital chaplain?

Ideally, these questions will not be used in interview fashion, one right after the other. The most appropriate use of the questions is as responses to verbal and nonverbal cues given by a patient which indicate he has spiritual concerns. There are times (such as in Case 14 on p. 72) when a nurse may want to use questions such as those found in Table 1 as an interview to focus on the patient's spiritual needs. Several questions could also be inserted into the nursing history taken on admission. Some health-care facilities have officially incorporated questions about spiritual needs into their nursing history format.[5] It can be especially helpful at the time of admission to the hospital to ask the patient if his pastor knows he is in the hospital, and if not, whether he would like to have him notified. If the hospital has a staff of chaplains available, the patient should be informed of their services and how to obtain them.

Spiritual crisis can occur for various reasons. By assessing the duration and etiology of a patient's spiritual needs, a nurse can more effectively plan to meet them. Long-term spiritual needs can be a precipitating factor in illness; however, illness may also be a precipitating factor in spiritual crisis. Physical pain can be the all-consuming focus of a patient's attention which clouds his or her perception of God's intervention in his or her life. Psychological distress may become so severe that a patient's relationship with God is drastically affected and his concept of God distorted. A sterile, impersonal environment, such as an intensive care unit, in which a person is cut off from significant relationships and made dependent on machines, may also create critical spiritual needs. Plans for spiritual care need to be made in view of the patient as a whole person, considering all his needs.

Planning

If one of the goals of total patient care is to assist the patient in establishing and/or maintaining a dynamic, personal relationship with God, then we need to identify those factors which are necessary to achieve that goal. Assessing and identifying spiritual needs does not complete a nurse's responsibility.

Spiritual care requires careful planning. When a nurse is already feeling the pressure of too much to do in too little time, the added burden of planning for spiritual care may seem unrealistic. Yet there are occasions when not meeting spiritual needs consumes more time and energy than it would take to meet them.

Case 11. Dr. Jacobs was a Protestant minister who was frequently readmitted with complications of carcinoma of the colon. During previous hospitalizations he was a kind, gentle man who talked freely about his faith. On his final admission he seemed to be a different person. He was in severe pain, was constantly nauseated and vomiting, and at times behaved irrationally. The night before he died, he was extremely restless and began to behave violently, striking as the nurse attempted to change his linen. He would throw his full emesis basin across the room each time he vomited. After the fourth bout of cleaning up the patient and the room, the nurse put a hand on his shoulder and said, "I'm going to pray for you, Dr. Jacobs. . . . Lord, I pray that you will comfort Dr. Jacobs. Give him your peace in this difficult time, strength to bear the pain, and the knowledge of your loving presence with him." After the prayer he became rational and relaxed. He thanked the nurse and spent a good evening visiting with his family. He slept through the night without vomiting or needing sedation, and died peacefully the next morning. ■

Meeting spiritual needs does not necessarily mean sitting down with a patient for extended periods of time, although that may be appropriate in some situations. It does mean setting goals for spiritual care *whenever* patient contact takes place. An ideal time to assess and meet spiritual needs is during morning and evening care. Not only is the nurse in the room for a good length of time, but the nurse is already communicating caring through touch while giving a bath or a backrub. It is a time when neither the nurse nor the patient is as uncomfortable with silence as at other moments since there are physical tasks to be accomplished. The patient may need that silence to let his thoughts develop without the fear of losing his audience if he stops talking. He knows the nurse will probably stay in his room until the tasks are completed.

Even when spiritual care appears to be crisis intervention, as it was with Dr. Jacobs, planning is important. The nurse chose to pray with Dr. Jacobs, rather than to call the doctor about increasing his sedation, because the nurse had already established that prayer was meaningful to him. Part of the nurse's long-range plan of care for Dr. Jacobs was to assist him in maintaining his relationship with God. When the crisis arose, the nurse was prepared to meet it from a spiritual perspective as well as a physical one.

Responsible planning of nursing care requires planning for continuity and for communication with other members of the health team.

Case 12. Mr. Evans was a seventy-five-year-old man, admitted for cataract surgery. He was accustomed to reading the Bible every night at home but was unable to do so after his eyes were dilated. When the medicine nurse came to give him his sleeping pill, he refused it. She replied, "But you didn't sleep at all last night!" He told her that if he could only read his Bible he'd sleep just fine. The nurse picked up his Bible from the bedside stand and asked Mr. Evans what he would like her to read. He requested a psalm, which she read to him. He slept well that night. The nurse then wrote on the Kardex, "h.s. sedation: read Bible to pt." ■

Case 13. Mrs. Sampson was a sixty-nine-year-old woman with terminal carcinoma. She had a strong faith, and according to her pastor, she had been a source of strength to him and other members of his church through the years. In the course of her illness she began to feel agitated, alone and depressed. God seemed very far away, and that frightened her. A nurse on the evening shift offered to pray with Mrs. Sampson and her spirits raised considerably. Realizing the value of prayer to Mrs. Sampson, the nurse wrote on the nursing care plan in the Kardex:

Pt. has been deeply religious, but she feels that God is far away from her at this time	Pray with pt. PRN

A student on the night shift and an R.N. on the day shift read the care plan and began to pray with the patient when she became agitated. Mrs. Sampson began to feel relaxed and secure because on each shift there was one nurse who could assist her spiritually. ■

The nursing care plan should outline the patient's needs with appropriate nursing measures to meet them. Spiritual needs should routinely be assessed and recorded.

Planning for a patient's spiritual care should also include an evaluation of who would be the most appropriate person to meet his or her spiritual needs. If a patient needs in-depth spiritual counseling, a clergy referral would be in order if the patient consents. Assignment of nursing personnel should be made with consideration of which nurse could best meet a patient's needs. If a patient needs spiritual intervention, a nurse who is sensitive to spiritual needs and able to intervene should be assigned to that patient.

Involvement with spiritual needs is an essential aspect of responsible nursing care. It cannot be the private project of one nurse. Spiritual needs should be included when patient care is discussed in team conferences and change-of-shift reports. Spiritual needs outlined in the nursing care plan should be reflected in the nurses notes so that effects of spiritual intervention can be evaluated. Spiritual care is too important to be carried out haphazardly. It must be thoughtfully planned, implemented and evaluated.

Implementing

The next step in the nursing process is to implement the plans that have been made. In doing this we must keep in mind two principles of spiritual intervention.

First, each patient is a unique individual with diverse needs. Meeting spiritual needs is a complex process. We cannot compile a list of standing orders for spiritual care. Each patient's needs must be carefully assessed. Although there are no pat answers, there is a clear focus. That focus is God, and the patient's relationship with him.

Second, to meet spiritual needs nurses need to evaluate their own relationship with God. Nurses who feel alienated from God or doubt his involvement in people's lives will find it difficult, if not impossible, to assist a patient spiritually. We need to be experiencing an ever-maturing trust relationship with God ourselves in order to assist a patient to establish and/or maintain a dynamic, personal relationship with God. Nurses who do not feel qualified to provide spiritual care have the responsibility to refer a patient with spiritual needs to someone who is able to intervene.

Perhaps here we should talk about a concern that often arises among Christian nurses. If a nurse believes that a person can only experience a dynamic personal relationship with God through confessing faith in Jesus Christ as Lord and Savior, can that nurse really meet spiritual needs if a patient does not profess that faith?

Perhaps this question can best be answered with an analogy. If a patient is terminally ill, can we still meet physical needs? Of course, we can and we must! The ideal goal of nursing care is to restore a patient to

full health and life. If this goal is unrealistic, however, we do not reduce
our efforts to make a person comfortable and maintain maximum functioning. For instance, a person with terminal cancer may have an infected
wound which requires weeks of dressing changes, irrigations and appli-
cations of medication. We conscientiously perform these procedures
even though we know they will not cure the cancer.

In the same way, we can enable a person to hear about God's love
and concern for him, and to experience God's presence to some degree,
even though he never does enter into a life-giving relationship with God
through faith in Jesus Christ. At times we may well play an important
role in assisting a patient to establish a lasting faith relationship with God,
but we cannot expect to convert every patient to faith in Christ anymore
than we expect ourselves to cure every patient of physical disease.

The nurse has four major resources available for meeting spiritual
needs: (1) the use of self, (2) the use of prayer, (3) the use of Scripture
and (4) referral to clergy. Each of these resources and principles for their
use will be expanded in the following chapters.

Evaluating

Evaluating nursing intervention is imperative if quality care is to be maintained. To evaluate, the cycle of the nursing process is repeated, this time
in the light of former observations and interpretations, goals set in planning, and the measures taken to achieve those goals. (See Figure 7.)
Again, the nurse observes the patient's affect and behavior to determine
whether change has taken place. Then the meaning of the change is interpreted to determine whether the goals set have been achieved and
whether they were appropriate. Further intervention can then be
planned around the effectiveness and appropriateness of the evaluated
nursing actions and patient responses.

If clear goals with measurable criteria were formulated in the planning
stage, evaluation will follow logically and easily. But criteria may be difficult to establish, especially when a nurse first begins to intervene spiritually. For example, a nurse may discern a spiritual need in an agitated
patient and decide that prayer would be an appropriate nursing action.
The nurse's goal might be "to communicate God's love and concern to
the patient," with the criteria for achievement being "the patient will

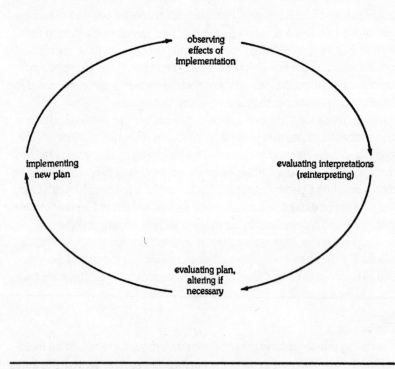

Figure 7. Evaluating in the Nursing Process

verbalize an awareness of God's concern and be able to rest calmly." After the nurse prays with the patient he breaks into tears. Has the nurse failed? Perhaps so. On the other hand, the communication of God's love to the patient may have uncovered feelings of guilt and worthlessness which were the cause of his agitation. Rather than giving up in defeat, the nurse will need to assess the meaning of the tears and plan appropriate intervention in the light of this unexpected development.

Perhaps it would be helpful to consider how a person looks and feels when his spiritual needs are met. Basically, we can expect him to look like a normal, relatively healthy person. He is not always calm and peaceful but experiences emotions appropriate to his situation. He has a strong and realistic self-image, warm and open interpersonal relationships, a sense of mission in life, and a confident trust-relationship with God.

If a person has had a strong faith prior to hospitalization and experiences only acute spiritual needs related to his illness, a realistic criterion for spiritual intervention might be "the patient will experience spiritual well-being." In most cases, however, "spiritual well-being" (that is, the result of a dynamic, personal relationship with God) is an overall goal, not a criterion. A person who has chronic, deeply rooted spiritual needs will require long-term care spiritually. Realistic criteria for beginning spiritual intervention for such a patient might be (1) that spiritual needs have been responsibly assessed and (2) that the chaplain has been called and is functioning as an integral member of the health-care team.

Because we are functioning as responsible members of the health-care team, when we intervene spiritually the patient's responses should be recorded in the nurse's notes. For example:

date and time	remarks	P.R.N.—medication underscored
10 PM	Pt. complained of severe pain unrelieved by <u>Demerol</u> <u>100 mg</u> given at 9 PM, appears agitated & tense. Pt. requested prayer. I prayed with her, after which she appeared to relax & stated that the pain was "easing."	
11 PM	Pt. sleeping.	
	G. Moore, R.N.	

Consistent recording of spiritual intervention and patient responses will provide an objective resource for long-term evaluation.

Nursing Standards

Criteria for spiritual well-being may also be expressed in terms of nursing standards. The following standard was developed by Roberta Lyder Paige, R.N., M.S.N., for use in a hospice program.

Outcome Standards for Hospice Nursing Practice: Spirituality

A. *Standard*

The client and family maintain or improve their level of spiritual health.

B. *Rationale*

1. Individuals are physical, psychosocial and spiritual beings.

2. Spiritual health affects psychosocial and physical health.

3. The spiritual needs for love and relatedness, meaning and forgiveness are more apparent in persons near death.

4. The extent to which an individual's spiritual needs are met directly affects his or her ability to cope with the dying process.

C. *Outcome Criteria*

The client and family:

1. report that their relationship with God has been maintained or improved;

2. demonstrate a hopeful attitude;

3. make use of appropriate religious ministrations including pastoral counseling, attendance at religious services, reading Scripture and religious literature, prayer, reconciliation (confession), anointing or laying on of hands with prayer;

4. maintain contact with those who have offered spiritual support and guidance in the past.

The Process in Action

When the nursing process is spelled out step-by-step, it seems cumbersome. Nurses often complain about being forced to take time to systematically plan and evaluate patient care. But in nursing practice the process flows smoothly and logically once a nurse becomes accustomed to functioning by it. Let us follow two patients through the nursing process to assess and meet their spiritual needs. Mr. Smith, Case 14, was a long-term patient with spiritual needs which lay far below the surface. Mrs. Henderson, Case 15, was admitted repeatedly for short intervals. At most times she demonstrated a strong faith which was a source of stability for her; however, during one hospitalization she faced a spiritual crisis.

Case 14. Mr. Smith, a fifty-one year-old man who became paraplegic six years ago after a diving accident, was admitted to a semi-private room with a diagnosis of chronic pyelonephritis and decubitus ulcers of the right hip. He seldom had visitors during the week. His wife visited only on Sundays and was always accompanied by other people. Visits by Mr. Smith's daughters, ages eighteen and twenty-one, always appeared strained. Both the daughters and Mr. Smith would sit silently staring at the floor. After each visit Mr. Smith would turn his head toward the wall and feign sleep. The pastor of Mr. Smith's church visited once a month. The pastoral visits appeared lighthearted and congenial, usually closing with a brief prayer offered by the pastor.

No flowers, cards, photographs or other personal effects decorated Mr. Smith's room. He was seldom demanding, but if his needs were neglected for any length of time he would respond cynically. He did have a television in his room. He occasionally watched sports, but he declared all other programs a waste of time.

Mr. Smith had some very real difficulties in his relationships with other people. To most of the nursing personnel he communicated only his most pressing needs. He answered their questions simply by yes or no. With one of the nurses he became quite verbal. This nurse listened sensitively, and he talked freely about his past, his family, his hopes and his fears.

The nurse involved with Mr. Smith thought about his relationships and began to question the meaning they held for him. "How does a nurse begin to meet Mr. Smith's spiritual needs? His relationships with people seem to be a fairly usualy mixture of warm, supportive friendships and the strained, difficult interactions, with perhaps the majority of the relationships being strained and difficult. How can I move from observing this rather unremarkable data to planning spiritual intervention?"

One Sunday evening, after visiting hours, Mr. Smith appeared to be unusually depressed. When the nurse came into his room, he was lying in bed with his face to the wall. He opened his eyes slightly to acknowledge the nurse's presence but said nothing. The nurse attempted to encourage Mr. Smith to verbalize his feelings about his relationships:

Ns: You seem sad since your visitors left, Mr. Smith.

Pt: That was my wife and daughters. The older one is married; that guy with her is her husband. They're so irresponsible! They don't know how to take care of themselves and they're going to have a baby already. The younger girl is a mess too. She lives at home, but she's out most of the time with her boyfriend and won't help around the house. My wife just had knee surgery and can't get around too well yet. I get so angry!

Ns: You feel sort of out of control?

Pt: That describes it exactly! I don't feel like I have control of my children—I can't do anything. And sitting in a wheelchair everyone has to look down on me . . . they used to look up to me. I was a tall man, 6'3". When I first landed in the wheelchair I thought there was no option but to kill myself . . . but I don't think about that anymore.

Ns: What made the difference?

Pt: My wife. I realized she needed me.

The nurse observed several significant results from this encounter with Mr. Smith. First, the goal of encouraging the patient to verbalize his feelings had been met as he expressed his feelings of anger and impotence as well as the importance his wife held for him. Another result which was perhaps more important was the new level of rapport the nurse established with Mr. Smith. By accurately interpreting his feelings the nurse was able to communicate to him an ability to hear what he was saying and an active concern. The nurse was then able to become a catalyst as Mr. Smith used his time in the hospital to re-evaluate who he was and where he was going in his life.

(To clearly differentiate the steps of the nursing process which have taken place in this interaction, we can put them in our diagram of the nursing process, as seen in Figure 8. The nursing process becomes a cycle. As we carry out our plan of action new information is obtained. The steps of observing and interpreting become an evaluation of the effectiveness and appropriateness of our nursing intervention.)

On further investigation Mr. Smith's relationship with his wife was found to be quite good. She visited so seldom because she was unable to drive due to recent surgery on her knees. She had to rely on friends and neighbors for transportation. She called twice a day, though, and was a tremendous support to Mr. Smith. Mr. Smith felt quite secure in his role as husband, seeing his relationship with his wife as being much

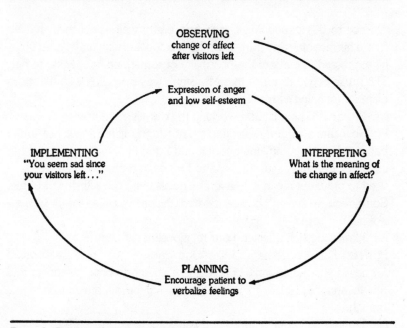

Figure 8. The Nursing Process in Case 14

deeper than a merely sexual one. She also seemed satisfied with their relationship.

Mr. Smith felt very inadequate in his role of father, however. He felt he had lost control of his children as they had gone through their teen-age years. He tried to maintain his role of disciplinarian in the family but felt helpless to follow through as he sat in his wheelchair with the children "looking down" at him. Mr. Smith was also frustrated about his relationship with his pastor, who seemed to have difficulty carrying on a serious conversation with him. The pastor's efforts to cheer him up only made Mr. Smith more miserable.

Mr. Smith seemed to remain in a state of emotional equilibrium until the third month of his hospitalization. His physical condition stayed fairly stable with very slow but steady progress toward healing. After the third month he became extremely depressed and stopped communicating with anyone, except to ask for basic needs to be met. At times he did not even request the urinal or bedpan and became incontinent for the first time since his admission.

Prior to this period Mr. Smith had pretty well established that he found his meaning and purpose in his relationship with his wife. At times he expressed fear about the possibility of something happening to her. The nurse began to sense that Mr. Smith was struggling with the more ultimate meaning of his life.

Ns: Mr. Smith, how is God working in your life right now?

Pt: Now that's a funny question... not funny like a joke, but funny because I've been thinking about it and I don't know the answer. I believe in God, and Jesus Christ, and I've been a pretty decent fellow. I used to pray, but recently I haven't. I guess that's the selfish part of me. Some requests haven't been answered, things I've asked for for years— not all, but some.

Ns: Has being sick affected your relationship with God?

Pt: Yes, I feel discouraged, like God doesn't hear me. I've prayed for healing but here I am a cripple and it's getting worse. I've never told this to anyone, not even Pastor Jones. My beliefs haven't changed, though.

Ns: Do you feel your faith in God is helpful to you?

Pt: Definitely yes! If it weren't for him, I'd be in worse shape. Just because he hasn't healed me... Sometimes I think the Dear Lord puts people on this earth to test them to see what they can endure. I guess he does care. I'm a lot better off than I could be. I need someone to give me a good talking to!

Ns: You get angry with God, then feel bad about it.

Pt: Yes, lying here in this hsopital bed I get to dwelling on myself and my problems and lose perspective. It helps to talk about it like this.

The conversation continued in this vein for about fifteen minutes. During that time Mr. Smith shared freely his feelings about himself and God. Although the nurse did not consistently pick up Mr. Smith's feelings accurately and sometimes asked questions that could have been diversionary, a listening attitude and concern about his spiritual needs stimulated him to think and to verbalize. Toward the end of the conversation Mr. Smith again brought up his feelings of guilt over not praying. The nurse asked him if he would like prayer for the things they had discussed. He agreed with enthusiasm. So the nurse prayed, "Heavenly Father, thank you that you remain with us even when we don't sense your presence. Thank you that you forgive us when we turn away from you and that you always draw us back into your love. Thank you for your love and concern for Mr. Smith, and for the fact that you understand his anger and frustration. We pray that you would strengthen and encourage him in this difficult time and keep him ever mindful of your presence with him. In Jesus' name. Amen."

Mr. Smith repeated the "Amen" affirmatively and lay back on the pillow, closing his eyes. He appeared relaxed and peaceful. "That really means a lot to me," he said smiling. "Thank you. You'll never know how much this means."

Mr. Smith made radical physical improvement in the next few weeks. His decubiti healed completely and his kidney infection cleared up. He began to sit in his wheelchair for longer and longer periods of time. His relationships with his family, visitors and staff improved. He came to the conclusion that he no longer needed to control his children. Their visits became a source of joy for him. He called his pastor and requested a private talk. They had their first serious conversation since Mr. Smith's accident.■

With his spiritual needs met, Mr. Smith was becoming free to live in harmony with God, himself and others. He could function as a whole person, in spite of his paraplegia.

Case 15. Mrs. Henderson sat cheerfully perched in her bed reading the Bible or devotional books most of the time. She was surrounded by religious cards and bouquets of flowers. She was a widow. Her only daughter lived in Germany with her serviceman husband, but Mrs. Henderson was surrounded by many warm and supportive friends. She was deeply involved with church work and served as a hospital volunteer. Daily she made rounds to all the other patients on the unit, filling water pitchers and spreading cheer.

On this admission Mrs. Henderson was to receive radiation therapy for carcinoma of the bladder following several transurethral resections in the past few years. When the nurse arrived with a wheelchair to take Mrs. Henderson to receive her first treatment, the patient had tears in her eyes, although she maintained a smile. The nurse sat down in the wheelchair beside Mrs. Henderson and said:

Ns: You seem upset.

Pt: Oh, it's just a silly thing.

Ns: But not too silly to be very upsetting to you. Are you concerned about the radiation therapy?

Pt: Yes, but I know I shouldn't be. Dr. Harris said the side effects would be minimal, and that it will slow the growth of the cancer.

Ns: But it's still frightening.

Pt: My husband died of cancer of the brain five years ago. He had radiation treatments for it and it was awful! He made me promise that if I ever had cancer, that I wouldn't let them give me any radiation. He eventually became like a vegetable. I guess I'm reliving that experience. I feel like I'm betraying my husband by going to radiation therapy, yet intellectually I know it would be foolish not to. I know my case is different. I've prayed about it and I feel that I should have the treatments, but I can't help feeling so alone.

Ns: There's a psalm that has meant a lot to me in the past. It's Psalm 16. [Picking up the patient's Bible from the bedside stand and reading] "I keep the LORD always before me; because he is at my right hand, I shall not be moved. Therefore my heart is glad, and my soul rejoices; my body also dwells secure."

Pt: [Taking the Bible and underlining the phrase "my body also dwells secure"] That's beautiful! It's just what I needed to know.

Ns: Would you like me to pray with you before we go downstairs?

Pt: Oh! Would you!

Ns: Father, you know how hard it is for Mrs. Henderson to go to radiation therapy today, and you understand how alone she feels. Thank you that you will go with her and that her body is secure in your hands. We praise you for your faithfulness to us. In Jesus' name. Amen.

Pt: Thank you, Lord, for sending your ministering angel to me. You do provide in strange and wonderful ways. Amen. [Turning toward the nurse] Okay, I'm ready to go to radiation therapy now. I feel it's the right thing to do.

(If we were to diagram this interaction it would look like Figure 9.)

Mrs. Henderson was discharged with some improvement but was soon readmitted for recurrent bladder tumors. Before she went to the operating room for another transurethral resection, the nurse who came with her preoperative injections asked, "Is there anything else I can do for

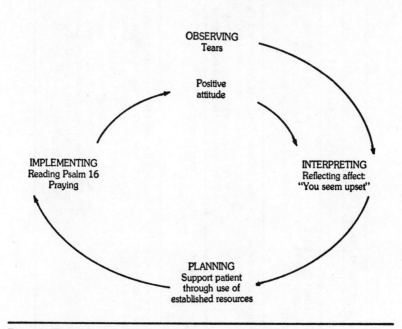

Figure 9. The Nursing Process in Case 15

you?" Mrs. Henderson replied, "Yes, there is. Would you pray with me please?" The nurse prayed with Mrs. Henderson and continued the spiritual support postoperatively.

Mrs. Henderson died several months later. After Mrs. Henderson's death, her daughter wrote a letter to the director of nursing commending the nursing staff. She said that what her mother had appreciated most was the prayer and spiritual encouragement of the nurses. ■

Including spiritual care in the nursing process contributes to quality care of the whole person. (Tables 2, 3 and 4 summarize how this may be done.)

Making a Nursing Diagnosis

In 1973 a movement began among nurses to develop a uniform system of labeling nursing problems. In many ways it has been a "grass roots" movement; it has not been sponsored by any major nursing organization. It has included nursing educators, theorists and practioners who

Table 2. *Meaning and Purpose: A Summary of Spiritual Needs and the Nursing Process*

	Observing	Interpreting	Planning & Implementing
1.	Does the patient have an illness which will affect his or her job, role as spouse or parent, living situation, community involvement?	What meaning does the patient place on the ability to maintain these roles? Is he or she able to see alternatives?	Treat the patient with respect and dignity. Help him to think through alternatives and to consider where his values lie.
2.	How does the patient spend his or her time in the hospital?	Can the patient make constructive use of time under the handicap of being in the hospital?	Present the patient with opportunities available at the hospital, such as occupational therapy, chapel services, representatives of "ostomy clubs," religious radio and television programs.
3.	Does his or her conversation and affect express hope or despair?	On what is his or her hope, or lack of hope, founded? Does God provide meaning and purpose for the patient?	Use question technique.
4.	Does the patient show any evidence of religious commitment (Bible reading, religious medals, asking for chaplain or pastor, prayer before meals)?	Does he or she gain hope from these practices? Does the patient feel God is listening, or does he feel alienated from God?	Encourage the faith the patient has through praying with the patient, reading and discussing appropriate Bible passages, talking about his or her relationship with God (and/or your own —but without preaching!). Help the patient secure anything necessary for the practice of his faith (Bible, rosary, prayer books, clergy). Family and chaplain's office should be able to provide these items.

Table 3. *Love and Relatedness: A Summary of Spiritual Needs and the Nursing Process*

	Observing	Interpreting	Planning and Implementing
1.	Who visits? How often? What is the atmosphere of the visits? What is the patient's affect and behavior after visitors leave?	Does a lack of visitors mean that the patient has no friends or family, or are there transportation problems, illness at home or similar difficulties? Can the patient be honest with visitors? Are his or her visitors supportive? Does his or her pastor visit? How does the patient feel about these visitors and visits?	Encourage the patient by your presence. Show empathy. Facilitate communication with family, friends, clergy. Encourage the patient to verbalize both positive and negative feelings about relationships. Reinforce God's love and concern for patient through prayer. Use of appropriate Scripture. Touch.
2.	What is the patient's behavior toward personnel?	Does the behavior reflect his true feelings, or is he either acting as he thinks he is expected to behave ("good patient") or redirecting fear and anger toward personnel?	
3.	What is the patient's behavior toward other patients, especially roommates? Does he isolate himself or reach out to other patients?	Does hospital behavior follow the usual pattern of patient's interpersonal relationships, or does it present a radical change? Has the patient's perception of other people's concern for him or her changed?	
4.	What articles are in the patient's room (cards, flowers, gifts, photos, religious books or objects)?	What meaning do the articles have to the patient?	
5.	What is the patient's affect?	Is it appropriate? Does affect correspond with what the patient is verbalizing?	

Table 4. Forgiveness: A Summary of Spiritual Needs and the Nursing Process

...ving	Interpreting	Planning and Implementing
1. Does the patient make comments like, "God is punishing me." "What did I do to deserve this?" "Why me?"	What is the patient's concept of God? (Does his God forgive?)	Listen empathetically without moralizing or offering platitudes.
2. Does the patient express anger or an unforgiving attitude toward friends or family? Is he cynical?	What does the patient's anger or cynicism mean? Does he need forgiveness from other people? Can he accept himself?	Help the patient to verbalize anger and identify source of guilt.
3. Is he or she depressed, withdrawn?	What is the source of the depression?	Encourage with presence, touch, empathy.
4. Is he or she either uncooperative or extremely cooperative?	Is the patient feeling guilty and either turning his anger with himself toward others or attempting to earn forgiveness by good works?	Encourage verbalization. If guilt is expressed, help the patient deal with its source. Refer if indicated.
5. Does he or she joke about heaven and hell or other religious topics?	Does joking reflect the patient's fear or anxiety about the afterlife?	Be certain the patient is not expressing serious concerns before laughing at his jokes.
6. Does he confess thoughts or actions of which he is ashamed?	What is the meaning of this confession?	Encourage the patient to confess to God. Communicate God's forgiveness through prayer, Scripture, own attitude toward patient. May need clergy referral for complex problem. The patient may desire communion.

attended the National Conferences on Classification of Nursing Diagnosis (held in 1973, 1975, 1978 and 1980) at their own initiative and expense.

The concept of nursing diagnosis is still in the development stage. There is not yet a final consensus about what the classifications should be, or even full agreement about the definition of a nursing diagnosis. The nursing theorists' group at the 1978 Conference contended that "Nursing diagnosis is a concise phrase or term summarizing a cluster of empirical indicators representing patterns of unitary man."[6] "Unitary man" is the theorists' model of human nature, which they would like to see accepted as *the* model for all nursing theory. The practicing nurses at the third Conference defined nursing diagnosis as "a diagnostic classification system for the purpose of directing nursing theory."[7]

In actual practice, the nursing diagnosis is a short statement describing what a nurse has assessed as a patient problem within the realm and

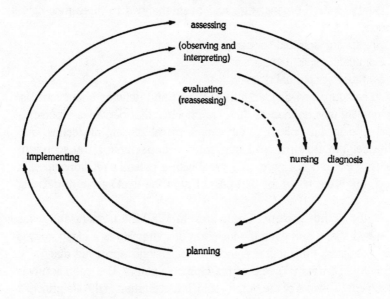

Figure 10. Nursing Diagnosis and the Nursing Process

responsibility of nursing. It fits into the nursing process at the conclusion of the assessment phase and forms the basis of planning and implementation (see Figure 10).

A nursing diagnosis is composed of two parts. First there is a statement preceded by "alteration in," "potential alteration in," or "dysfunction in." These terms describe functional behaviors which facilitate health. The second part of the statement is preceded by "related to" and describes the problems a nurse can work with to restore or maintain health.[8] The first category which described spiritual needs, proposed in 1973, was "Alteration in Faith in God."[9] Using that classification, a nursing diagnosis for a person who feels alienated from God because of intense, prolonged suffering could be "Alteration in Faith in God Related to Suffering." But such a diagnosis is not functional, because a nursing diagnosis should provide enough data to begin treatment. Perhaps with further assessment, a diagnosis could be made of "Alteration of Faith in God Related to Anger at God Over Suffering."

By 1978 the nomenclature had been changed to three new categories:

Spirituality: spiritual concern
Spirituality: spiritual distress
Spirituality: spiritual despair

Each category was divided into etiologies and defining characteristics. Spirituality was defined as "the life principle that pervades a person's entire being, his volitional, emotional, moral-ethical, intellectual, and physical dimensions, and generates a capacity for transcendent values."[10] It did not necessarily deal with a person's relationship with God, but it did allow for that possibility in the etiologies and defining characteristics.

At the Fourth National Conference in 1980 the nomenclature was changed again, and even the inclusion of spirituality as a category was hotly debated. Finally, it was included as a single approved diagnosis, "Spiritual Distress (Distress of the Human Spirit)." The definition was modified: "Distress of the human spirit is a disruption in the life principle which pervades a person's entire being and which integrates and transcends one's biological and psychosocial nature."[12] The etiologies and defining characteristics were sharply reduced.

Table 5. Nursing Diagnosis of Spirituality—1978[11]

I. Spiritual Concerns
Etiology
Challenged belief system
Separation from religious cultural ties
Anticipated role change
Concerned about relationship with
    God
Unresolved feelings about the concept
    of death
Search for more meaning or purpose
    in existence
Disrupted religious practices
Defining Characteristics
Investigates various beliefs
Verbalizes inner conflict about beliefs
Questions credibility of religious cul-
    tural system
Discouraged
Mild anxiety
Bewildered
Anticipatory grief
Questions meaning for own existence
Concern about relationship with God/
    deity
Unable to participate in usual religious
    practices, i.e., daily prayers,
    Communion, meditation, worship
    services
Attempts to substitute simplified rituals
    in place of usual worship
Unable to obtain specific foods re-
    quired by faith/belief system

II. Spiritual Distress
Etiology
Separation from religious cultural ties
Challenged belief and value system
Sense of meaninglessness/purpose-
    lessness
Remoteness from God
Disrupted spiritual trust
Moral-ethical nature of therapy

Sense of guilt/shame
Intense suffering
Unresolved feelings about death
Anger toward God
Defining Characteristics
Common to All Etiologies
(One of the following must be present)
Struggling with meaning in life/death
Seeks spiritual assistance
Disturbance in concepts/perception
    of God or belief system
Disturbance in sleep/rest pattern
Moderate to severe anxiety
Crying
Varying degrees of grieving
Depression
Preoccupation
Psychosomatic manifestations
Degrees of anger
Degrees of guilt
Defining Characteristics
Related to the Above
Specific Etiologies
*Separation from Religious Cultural
Ties*
    Loneliness
    Sense of powerlessness
    Doubts credibility of religious
        cultural system
Challenged Belief and Value System
    Ambivalent about own and others'
        belief systems
    Difficulty in receiving assistance
*Sense of Meaninglessness/Purpose-
lessness*
    Cynicism
    Considers suicide
    Questions meaning in suffering
    Feelings of uselessness
    Withdrawal
    Apathy

Self-destructive behavior
Sexual activity disturbance
Remoteness from God
    Lacks a feeling of unity with God
    Sense of spiritual emptiness
    Gains little satisfaction in prayer
    Verbalizes that God seems very
        distant
    Verbalizes a desire to feel close
        to God
Disrupted Spiritual Trust
    Doubts compassion of superior
        being
    Worries about loss of trust
    Ambivalence
    Resentment
    Feelings of alienation
Moral-Ethical Nature of Therapy
    Sense of powerlessness (trapped
        feeling)
    Ambivalence in decisions
    Questions or refuses therapeutic
        regime
    Agrees to morally/ethically
        unacceptable therapy
    Frantic seeking of advice or support
        for decision making
Sense of Guilt/Shame
    Wish to undo, redo, relive the past
    Expression of shame, regret,
        sinfulness, guilt
    Bitterness, recrimination
    Inability to forgive self or receive
        forgiveness
    Views illness as punishment from
        God
    Doubts acceptance by God
    Self-belittling
    Projection of blame
    Self-destructive behavior
    Sexual activity disturbance

Intense Suffering
    Questions meaning of suffering
    Fear of ability to endure suffering
    Ambivalence toward God
    Questions credibility of God/belief
        system
    Expresses that suffering is
        necessary reparation
    Self-focus as demonstrated by
        withdrawal, irritability,
        restlessness, agitation, self-pity
        or fatigue
Unresolved Feelings about Death
    Fears (i.e., darkness, being alone,
        going to sleep, etc.)
    Concern about life after death
    Disturbing dreams
    "Gallows" humor
    Demanding behavior
    Avoidance/preoccupation with
        subject of death
Anger toward God
    Feels resentment, hostility,
    alienation
    Perceives illness as punishment
        from God
    Reluctance to participate in spiritual
        rituals
    Rebelliousness
    Displacement of anger toward
        religious representative

III. Spiritual Despair
Etiology
Self-disintegration
Lack of will to live
Lost belief in self
Lost belief in treatment
Lost belief in value system and/or God
Defining Characteristics
Hopelessness
Sense of meaninglessness

Loss of spiritual belief
Death wish (escapism)
Sense of exhaustion
Sense of abandonment
Sees no meaning in suffering
Requires extreme effort to function
Withdrawal
Severe depression
Loss of affect
Refusal to communicate with loved ones
Discontinued religious participation

Etiologies for Future Consideration with Defining Characteristics

Religious Immaturity
Unclear differentiation regarding beliefs/values ("I believe what I was taught")
Feels no freedom of religious choice
Persistent indecision about spiritual beliefs
Motivated by self-gratification
Verbalizes little about religious meaning in relation to health/illness
Excessive verbalization about spiritual relation to health/illness
No verbalization of feelings, acts and experiences related to belief system
Lack of integration; behavior incongruent with stated belief
Evidence of magical thinking
Uses religious themes to manipulate people
Dabbling in a variety of religious experiences
Inability to make commitment, closed to growth

Distorted View of Basic Religious Tenets
Guilt

Sees illness as punishment
Inadequate substitution of rituals

Unresolved Hostility toward a Particular Church, Religion, Religious Representative
Anger
Cynicism
Outburst
Refusal to accept visitation by religious representative

Group members who prepared the documents on "Matters of Spirituality" were:
Claire Campbell, Dallas, TX
Barbara Fisher, Toronto, Ontario
Becky Fleeger, Manhattan Beach, CA
Anne Kuempel, Austin, TX
Trudi McFarland, Oakton, VA
Eileen Otis, New Orleans, LA
Luella Penner, Hudson, WI
Marie Prince, Sault Ste. Marie, Ontario
Arlene Thompson, London, Ontario
Sr. Joyce Turnbull, San Francisco, CA
Judy Van Heukelem, San Bruno, CA
Eleanor Vogel, St. Paul, MN
Group facilitators were:
Maria Meyer, St. Louis, MO
Pat Stelzer, St. Louis, MO

Place: St. Louis, Missouri
Date: April 1978
Event: The Third Nursing Conference on Classification of Nursing Diagnosis

Reprinted from *The Nurses Lamp* 30, No. 1, September 1978.

Table 6. *Spiritual Distress (Distress of the Human Spirit)—1980*[13]

Etiology	Defining characteristics
Separation from religious/cultural ties Challenged belief and value system, e.g., due to moral/ethical implications of therapy, due to intense suffering	*Expresses concern with meaning of life/ death and/or belief systems Anger toward God Questions meaning of suffering Verbalizes inner conflict about beliefs Verbalizes concern about relationship with deity Questions meaning for own existence Unable to participate in usual religious practices Seeks spiritual assistance Questions moral/ethical implications of therapeutic regime Gallows humor Displacement of anger toward religious representatives Description of nightmares/sleep disturbances Alteration in behavior/mood evidenced by anger, crying, withdrawal, preoccupation, anxiety, hostility, apathy, etc.

*Critical defining characteristic

Those who would like to remove spirituality from the approved list of nursing diagnoses do not necessarily believe that spiritual needs are unimportant, but that they fall under other categories. Many of the approved categories do overlap and can become cumbersome, so work is still under way to reduce the number of categories and simplify the nursing diagnosis process.

"Spiritual Distress" does not seem to be an adequate category, for if we are defining nursing as health maintenance as well as restoration of health and supportive care until death, then nursing measures should prevent spiritual distress as well as treat it. However, even the "spiritual distress" diagnosis does provide numerous opportunities for spiritual nursing intervention. Spiritual distress can be related to each of the spiritual needs described previously.

Using the diagnosis of "spiritual distress" we can re-examine the case studies of Mr. Smith and Mrs. Henderson (pages 72-79). Mr. Smith, who was unable to participate in church functions because of his illness and was angry at God for his prolonged suffering, could be diagnosed as being in "spiritual distress related to separation from religious ties" and "spiritual distress related to a challenged belief system." Nursing care included reuniting Mr. Smith with his religious ties by involving his pastor, and reinforcing his belief system by allowing him to verbalize his feelings and praying with him.

Mrs. Henderson exhibited "spiritual distress related to a challenged belief and value system regarding the moral/ethical implications of therapy." She was experiencing conflict between what she believed was right and the promise she had made to her dead husband. By supporting her already strong faith, reinforcing it with a passage of Scripture and praying appropriately with her, the nurse enabled Mrs. Henderson to overcome her spiritual distress.

In many ways, nursing diagnosis is nothing new; it is merely a standardized form of saying what we have been doing all along. As with medical diagnoses, labels can be useful in communicating clearly what we mean. They can give us a concrete problem which can be fixed in a measurable way that enhances our accountability. However, standard nomenclature also holds its dangers. While it may define the practice of nursing, it may also limit its scope. The list of "approved" diagnoses should never be closed, or we may one day find ourselves in an extinct profession. Another danger is that although the various classifications of nursing diagnoses should alert us to considering the needs of the whole person, we may miss unique nursing problems which occur in patients whose needs do not fit into the standard categories.

Many schools of nursing are beginning to teach nursing diagnosis in their curricula. Some hospitals and health care agencies are using it in nursing care plans. Eventually, the concept of nursing diagnosis should provide a tool for clearer and more accurate communication among nurses and members of the health care team. It should eventually define nursing, but in the meantime nursing is still trying to define itself, so much work remains to be done.

Table 7: *Spiritual Distress Diagnosis*[14]
   SPIRITUAL DISTRESS RELATED TO
   NEED FOR LOVE AND RELATEDNESS

PHYSICAL/EMOTIONAL DISEQUILIBRIUM

Need to establish relationship
bewilderment
anxiety
alienation

Need to maintain relationship
loneliness
sense of abandonment

SPIRITUAL DISEQUILIBRIUM

Non-Verbal Behavior

investigates various beliefs
seeks spiritual assistance
frantically seeks advice or
   support for decisions

attempts to substitute simplified
   rituals in place of usual
   worship
seeks spiritual assistance

Anger toward God
reluctant to participate in
   spiritual rituals
rebels
displaces anger toward religious
   representative

Verbal Expressions

ambivalent about own and
   others' belief systems
verbalizes inner conflict about
   beliefs
questions credibility of religious-
   cultural system
doubts credibility of religious-
   cultural system
sense of spiritual emptiness

expresses concern about
   relation with God/deity
disturbance in concept/percep-
   tion of God or belief system
ambivalent toward God
questions credibility of God/
   belief system
doubts compassion of superior
   being

Remoteness from God
lacks a feeling of unity with God
feels spiritually empty
gains little satisfaction in prayer
verbalizes that God seems very
   distant
verbalizes desire to feel close
   to God

SPIRITUAL DISTRESS RELATED TO NEED FOR FORGIVENESS	SPIRITUAL DISTRESS RELATED TO NEED FOR MEANING AND PURPOSE	
	In life and death	*In suffering*
bitterness	fears (darkness, being alone, going to sleep, etc.)	self-focus (demonstrated by withdrawal, irritability,
recrimination	feelings of uselessness,	restlessness, agitation,
self-belittling	hopelessness,	self-pity, fatigue)
projection of blame	meaninglessness	feelings of hopelessness
	demanding behavior	feelings of powerlessness
	apathy, withdrawal	
	cynicism	
	loss of affect	
	depression	
	requires extreme effort to function	
	sense of exhaustion	
inability to forgive self or receive forgiveness	disturbing dreams	self-destructive behavior
self-destructive behavior	avoidance or preoccupation with subject of death	
	discontinued religious participation	
	self-destructive behavior	
	refusal to communicate with loved ones	
wish to undo, redo, relive the past	struggles with meaning in life and death	questions about meaning in suffering
expressions of shame, regret, sinfulness, guilt	questions about meaning of own existence	expression that suffering is necessary reparation
illness seen as punishment from God	concern about life after death	illness seen as punishment from God
doubts about acceptance by God	"gallows" humor	fear of ability to endure suffering
	loss of spiritual belief	
	death wish (escapism)	

Signs of physical/emotional disequilibrium possible in all needs

disturbance in sleep/rest pattern	grief
psychosomatic manifestations	crying
sexual activity disturbance	depression
discouragement	preoccupation
anxiety	anger

Chapter 5
The Use
of Self

They're Yours... These Hands

Praise You, Lord, for fashioned man
made from the simple dust

that from eternity
O God, You had

a plan,

A vessel... as You please to use
I praise You, Lord, for shaping me

marred, broken, mended, fired
restored. Could I

refuse?

I praise You, Lord, for love and zeal
You formed these outstretched hands. I pray

like Him, my loving touch

betimes, perhaps

may heal.

Elisabeth Fuller, R.N.

The therapeutic use of self is a practical reflection of the biblical view of man. In using ourselves therapeutically, we affirm that each patient is a person of value who is worthy of our time and involvement. This requires that we have a degree of self-understanding and a sense of self-worth which come from a relationship with God. Travelbee states, "To use oneself therapeutically also implies that the nurse possesses a profound understanding of the human condition. . . . The nurse realizes that her spiritual values, or her philosophical beliefs about human beings, illness and suffering will determine the extent to which she will be able to help others find meaning (or no meaning) in these situations."[1]

The therapeutic use of self implies that we relate to patients as individuals, person-to-person, without benefit of props. It is *being* as opposed to *doing*. It involves giving supportive presence to another human being. To effectively use ourselves therapeutically we must be willing to become both vulnerable and committed to another individual. It requires a humility which enables us to care for patients as fellow human beings rather than approaching them in the authority of the nurse role. It is not an easy task, for it demands a giving of ourselves to others which may leave us feeling drained. Frequently we avoid the therapeutic use of self to protect ourselves. One nurse observed this happening on a unit:

Just when the patients need us we are gone. Often not physically gone, but by cutting off communication we are not really there. We are not really hearing what they are saying to us by the constant buzzing of the buzzer, the cross words, the dissatisfaction. We convince the physician to order a sedative or a larger dose of pain medication—anything to keep them quiet—to keep us from going into the room. Anything to keep us from losing our professionalism, for if we stopped to listen, we might find that we are as incurably human as they. We might even have to say that we are afraid, or worse yet, we might even cry. That seems to be the epitome of going too far, of getting too involved.[2]

Listening, empathy, vulnerability, humility and commitment—the key elements in the therapeutic use of self—are skills which must be acquired through faith, education and practice. Romans 12:14-16 summarizes these functions in practical terms: "Bless those who persecute you; bless and do not curse them. Rejoice with those who rejoice, weep with those who weep. Live in harmony with one another; do not be haughty, but associate with the lowly; never be conceited."

This injunction from Romans goes beyond a mere idealistic "love for all humanity" and a desire to be helpful to a practical application of the belief that God created human beings in his own image. The source of strength in our ability to use ourselves therapeutically comes from God through our faith. Faith alone, however, does not create refined skills. Education and practice are necessary to give direction and substance to a faith-based desire to be helpful.

Listening

Listening is an acquired skill It involves hearing and understanding not only all of what people are saying but also what they are afraid to say. Listening carefully enables nurses to perceive some of the reasons behind patients' verbal communications.

At times we may fail to hear clear verbal expressions of a person's needs. There are unconscious barriers to listening which cause us to use *selective listening*—hearing only what we feel equipped to handle. As we become aware of these barriers, we can begin to overcome them and hear what our patients are really saying.[3] (See Figure 11.)

Word meanings may be a barrier to hearing a person's expression of spiritual needs. Each denomination and sect has a unique vocabulary for describing important aspects of faith and practice. For instance, the terms which define a person's faith relationship with God may differ. "Being a Christian," "becoming a believer," "getting saved," "being born again," "being baptized" and "awakening to new life in Christ" may seem synonymous to some people; to others only one of these terms

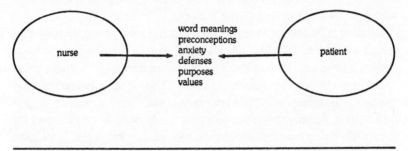

Figure 11. Barriers to Listening

may be accurate. Lingo may be a convenient shortcut in communication, but only if we are sure it means the same thing to a patient as it does to us.

Preconceptions prevent us from hearing clearly what others are saying. The most overriding preconception which forms a barrier in spiritual care is feeling that anyone who is truly serious about a relationship with God must believe what we believe and behave as we behave. For instance, we might feel that anyone who uses profanity could not possibly have spiritual concerns. As soon as a patient uses a profane word, it may ring so loudly in our ears that we cannot hear an expression of spiritual needs.

Anxiety creates a barrier to listening because it puts the focus on the nervous nurse rather than the patient and his needs. Any time we are faced with the demands of mastering new skills, anxiety over the task we are performing may prevent us from seeing the patient as a person. For this reason we may not become involved in meeting spiritual needs when we are engulfed by a new situation. Once we become comfortable with *ourselves* in a clinical area, we will be better able to hear our patient's expression of anxiety.

Closely related to anxieties are personal *defenses*. When a person offends us or attacks something we hold dear, we tend to put up defenses to protect ourselves and our values. For instance, a patient's expression of anger toward God might cause a nurse to respond by defending God rather than hearing the patient's cry of desperation. Another patient's seductive behavior might cause a nurse to avoid the patient rather than setting limits and listening to the patient.

While it is essential to set goals for nursing care, *purposes* may also create a barrier to listening. For instance, a nurse may begin to teach a patient how to care for a colostomy, but the patient says, "I'm not going to live long enough to bother with all that." The nurse, intent on teaching the procedure, responds, "Of course you will!" and continues to give instructions. Another common example is when we feel so pressed for time while giving medications that we cannot stop long enough to listen to a patient.

Finally, *values* prevent us from listening with open ears. We are constantly faced with patients whose values are different from our own. It is often difficult to have compassion for someone who has violated our own moral standards and suffered for it. We tend to think that person deserves what he got. For example, if a nurse feels that abortion is wrong, that nurse may be unable to listen compassionately to the fears and concerns of a woman undergoing the procedure.

All of us have certain values which govern our moral behavior. These values arise out of our beliefs, experiences and environment. When we force our values on other people, we unconsciously assume that their beliefs, experiences and environment are the same as our own. To suspend judgment so that we may listen to the hurts, fears and concerns of others may reveal that we too could have acted in a similar manner had we been subjected to the same influences. To listen with sensitivity does not require that we condone behavior which violates our moral values, but it does enable us to empathize with people. Through empathy we can become agents of creative change.

Empathy
Empathy is the ability to understand what a person is feeling and to communicate that understanding to him while remaining objective enough to see why he feels as he does and to be able to assist him. Empathy is a process involving both the intellect and the emotions. (See Figure 12.)

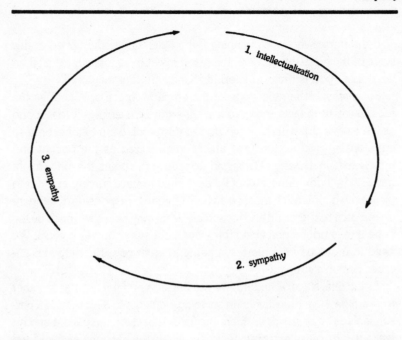

Figure 12. The Empathy Process

Intellectual consideration is the first stage of the process. It is basically the first step of the nursing process. It involves observation—collecting the facts about a patient's affect, behavior, diagnosis, environment and so on. If we stop at this stage, we do not come close to empathy, but remain aloof and tend to propose solutions which are not helpful.

Case 16.   Betty was an attractive twenty-five-year-old legal secretary who had bilateral silicone breast implants. She was single. Her boyfriend visited her after surgery and acted intimate toward her. He insisted on caressing her breasts in spite of the nurses' constant warning that infection might result. She was readmitted the week after discharge with severe infection in both breasts. The implants had to be removed and her surgeon recommended that they not be replaced. Betty went into a deep depression. Most of the nursing staff felt that Betty had brought her problems on herself, so they spent little time with her. Finally Betty broke into tears as a nurse was changing her dressing. "What am I going to do?" she asked. "My boyfriend likes women with big breasts. I suppose he'll leave me for someone else." ■

If the nurse who was changing Betty's dressing had stopped at this stage of the empathy process, the nurse might have replied, "Well then why didn't you tell him to keep his hands off your incisions?"

Sympathy is the next stage of the empathy process. We move the focus away from facts and onto feelings—our own feelings. We respond as if we were the patient. If we stop at this point, we might become so emotionally involved that we are as immobilized as the patient and unable to help. If Betty's nurse had stopped at this point, the nurse might have said, "I don't know what I'd do if I had to have surgery in order to please my boyfriend. It must be awful!" Our inner response is dependent on our own background and resources. What may be felt as a crisis by the patient may not be perceived this way by the nurse and vice versa. We need to move beyond mere sympathy to enter constructively into another person's struggle.

At the final stage, *empathy,* we put the facts and the feelings together to examine them objectively. In so doing we begin to discern why a person feels as he or she does. Here the focus is back on the patient and his feelings. The nurse can now begin to support the patient effectively and encourage him toward constructive action. An empathetic response from Betty's nurse might have been, "That must be very frightening." The progression of intellectual and emotional responses was:

1. Intellectual considerations: Betty looks frightened and depressed. Her implants have been removed and probably will not be replaced. She feels that having large breasts is essential to keep her boyfriend.

2. Sympathy: I don't know what I'd do if I were in Betty's situation. I'd be scared and depressed, too. I can't understand how a man can make his relationship with Betty depend on the size of her breasts. I'd hate him!

3. Empathy: If Betty's feelings are as ambivalent and as strong as mine would be, she probably needs to talk about them. If her boyfriend's opinion of her really is based on the size of her breasts, and she cared enough about him to have silicone implants, her self-image must be pretty low. She needs someone to reinforce her sense of worth as a person. She needs to know her worth in God's eyes.

The process of empathy becomes almost instantaneous in a sensitive, mature nurse; however, looking at the stages will enable us to discover where the difficulty lies if our responses do fall short of empathy. If we find ourselves remaining cool and aloof with patients, we should spend some time considering what barriers in our own emotions prevent us from entering into our patients' concerns. Thinking back on crises we have encountered, how we felt, and what kind of help we wanted at the time may increase our awareness of patients' feelings and needs. If we find ourselves overwhelmed by our concern for patients—we "take them home with us" and become depressed over their problems—we should spend more time looking at the objective facts, do some research on creative alternatives, and read books about people who have endured suffering and overcome serious handicaps to lead meaningful and productive lives.[4]

Vulnerability

The therapeutic use of self requires that a nurse be vulnerable. To "feel with" the patient opens us to the possibility that we too will experience pain. To offer ourselves as a resource to other people creates the likelihood that at some time we will be rejected. The use of self involves lending people our strength until they can regain their own strength. We may feel drained in the process.[5] Nurses who are vulnerable are those who are willing to open themselves up to rejection, criticism and pain, as well as to the joy and praise of other people, as they respond to these people in a caring relationship. Vulnerability means a willingness to share another person's experiences, as this nurse did with Mary:

Monday, June 1: *Today I was assigned to Mary again. She is a thirty-year-old mother of five children with intractable congestive heart failure. She has shared a great deal with me, and I with her, during the past month of her hospitalization. It has not been an easy experience, but I have learned so much.*

Mary has caused me to do a great deal of reflecting on the meaning and necessity for an active philosophy—a personal philosophy of commitment in caring for any patient, but especially the dying. I remember a quote from Marcel, "The person who is at my disposal is the one who is capable of being with me with the whole of himself when I am in need; while the one who is not at my disposal seems merely to offer me a temporary loan raised on his resources. For the one, I am a presence;

for the other, I am an object."[6]

Mary has voiced these sentiments throughout our relationship. I have not always been with her with "the whole of myself." She knows it. I know it. Yet Mary has helped me understand more clearly the meaning of the therapeutic use of self—that in order for me to be really therapeutic I must involve myself with my patients, not just communicating with them, but communing with them.

Communication, to me, means a simple transference of information given out by one person and received by another. Communion is more than that. Communion is an act of sharing, a receiving as well as a giving by both persons in the relationship. Communion is an exchange of ideas, thoughts, feelings and needs. It involves mutual understanding.

Am I willing to enter into all of my patients' needs and experiences or only those I feel most comfortable with? Am I willing to let myself become vulnerable to their suffering and pain by asking them to share their feelings with me? Communion implies intimacy. It happens when you allow yourself to be vulnerable and involved.

Tuesday, June 2: Mary died today. I feel stunned. It hurts.[7]

Allowing ourselves to be vulnerable is nothing more than a recognition of our humanity. As human beings we are vulnerable. We hurt, we are intimidated by death, we experience pain physically and emotionally—we need someone to support us as we support patients. To function as if we were not vulnerable is destructive to our personality structures, and unhelpful to our patients.

Humility

To recognize our own humanity is also an expression of humility. To know we are human is to recognize our limits as well as our strengths. Humility protects us from the temptation to feel omnipotent and indispensable. It enables us to trust others to care for our patients. The use of self can create a bond which causes us to feel we own our patients. At that point the use of self ceases to be therapeutic and becomes manipulative. It also becomes a barrier to teamwork and continuity of care. From a spiritual perspective, humility is the realization that God can use another nurse in a patient's life just as easily as he can use me.

Humility characterizes the nurse who approaches patients expecting to learn from them. If we think we know all there is to know about a patient, we will not be able to use ourselves therapeutically. We already have the patient figured out so our interaction with him will only serve to substantiate our previous conclusions. Thus, we treat the patient as an intellectual challenge rather than as a person to be known and respected.

Humility allows patients to be themselves. We care for them because of their own intrinsic worth, not because they meet our needs or society's needs. Humility demands that we give the same level of care and understanding to each patient regardless of his moral standards, socioeconomic level, or physical and mental condition.

Humility enables us to be ourselves. If we have no pretensions, we are not humiliated when others see us as we truly are, for the image we project is our real self. We are free to rejoice with those who rejoice, weep with those who weep. We are able to become involved with our patients and freely admit that we are as incurably human as they are.[8]

Commitment

Finally, if we are to use ourselves therapeutically, a degree of commitment is required. Sister Madeleine Clemence describes commitment as "the full, willing, and open-eyed acceptance of one's full share of life, with its love given and received, its hopes and its disappointments, its joys and its sorrows. It is the acceptance of the solitude, the anxiety, the suffering and, finally, the death, which are the common lot of man."[9]

More specifically, commitment is a willingness on our part to share in the solitude, anxiety, suffering and grief of our patients. When we use ourselves therapeutically to meet the spiritual needs of a patient, we have communicated a deep degree of commitment to that patient as a person of value by the very nature of our involvement. We must be willing to continue that level of relationship as long as the patient needs spiritual support.

To refuse to be committed to a patient after beginning to intervene spiritually can be compared to a lifeguard who says to a nonswimmer, "Come on into the water; it's safe; I'll hold you up," and then decides to take his lunch break as the person takes his first tentative steps into the water. The emotional energy expended by a patient who begins to express his spiritual needs can be great. He may have had to overcome tremendous emotional barriers to open himself to another person on such a deep level. If we refuse to continue our involvement, the patient may hesitate to mention his spiritual needs again, just as the nonswimmer may develop a fear of the water after the lifeguard disappoints him. Commitment means dealing responsibly and compassionately with the results of our intervention through the therapeutic use of self.

Ultimately, commitment is the reflection of God's relationship with humanity. When we meet spiritual needs through the therapeutic use of self, we often represent God to the patient. Our commitment, or lack of commitment, may determine a patient's perception of God's love. For that reason the use of self alone is insufficient in meeting spiritual needs. Our goal in spiritual care is to assist patients in establishing and maintaining a relationship with God. Our aim is to direct their dependence toward God rather than ourselves. To do so we need other resources beyond the therapeutic use of self. The use of prayer and Scripture place the focus on God as the source of strength and healing.

Chapter 6
The Use
of Prayer

Mrs. Dawson taught me a lot about prayer when I cared for her. One day I came into her room. She was in agony. There was little anyone could do for her from a physical standpoint. She asked me to sit down. After I sat for about five minutes she asked me to pray for her. I asked her what she wanted me to pray for. Her request was that the pain would go away.

It took me a few minutes to decide what to pray or even whether to pray. I was thankful Mrs. Dawson's eyes were closed so she couldn't see my struggle. I just didn't think God would do that for her. The pain was so intense. Medication could not control it. I also wondered what would happen to Mrs. Dawson's already weak faith if I prayed and the pain did not go away.

Finally I went ahead and prayed, asking God to forgive my lack of faith. I prayed that God would relieve Mrs. Dawson's pain and show her he really cared for her. Ten minutes later her pain was gone and Mrs. Dawson was asleep.

The pain returned the next day, but Mrs. Dawson and I had experienced the power of a personal God who meets us in our times of greatest need.

From the diary of an R.N.

Prayer is intimate conversation between us and God. It is our response to God's initiative. Prayer is a recognition of our human limitations and our need for God. In many ways it is a move out of the confusion of our situation toward a mature and steady hope.[1] True prayer is a dialog. It is openness to God's will as well as the statement of our requests, thoughts and feelings to God.

When we have a dynamic personal relationship with God, prayer is the vital lifeline in that relationship. Through prayer we receive perspective, power and the assurance of God's presence with us. The life and teachings of Jesus give us insight into the importance and meaning of prayer. He took time out of a busy schedule to be alone and pray (Mt. 14:23). He shared his personal agony with God the Father in prayer (Mt. 26:39). He interceded on behalf of those he loved (Jn. 17). He also prayed for his enemies as he taught his disciples to do (Lk. 23:34). He taught about God's generosity in response to prayer (Mt. 7:7-11), about the importance of coming to God humbly and simply (Mt. 8:1-13) and about the power of praying in unity with others (Mt. 18:19-20).

In the Acts of the Apostles and the letters of the New Testament we get a glimpse of the importance of prayer to the early Christians. We see prayer as a dynamic link with a powerful and personal God. Prayer is vital to the spiritual life of Christians.

Illness and crisis can create a barrier to personal prayer. The reason is usually that the patient's ability to sense God's presence becomes clouded by the intensity of the problem.

Case 17. Jerry Wells, a twenty-nine-year-old truck driver, was hospitalized with spinal injuries from an automobile accident. It was his second serious accident in six months. When he was informed of closed circuit TV chapel services on Sunday morning he replied, "I don't think the Man upstairs likes me anymore. We don't seem to be on speaking terms." Jerry had been active in church prior to the second accident.■

Case 18.   Mary Gowen, a twenty-five-year-old director of Christian education, became severely affected with colitis. She wrote in her diary, "My prayers don't seem to be getting through. I feel so selfish. I just keep dwelling on myself and praying for God to heal me. I can't seem to get beyond this point. I know God hears other people's prayers but he doesn't seem to hear me."■

Case 19.   Sarah Johnson, a seventy-nine-year-old grandmother who had always had a deep faith, confessed to a nurse, "God seems so far away right now. I don't understand it, but I can't seem to pray anymore."■

Many factors enter into the disruption of a person's ability to pray. The normal stages of grief affect a person's relationship with God as well as his relationships with other people. A patient may think God does not hear, does not care, or does not know about his concerns. He may blame God for his illness and feel angry toward God, then feel guilt over his anger. He may try to bargain with God, and then give up in despair. He may be so overwhelmed by his present situation that he thinks no one, including God, can help him. In any case, the patient *feels* he is not getting through to God. In Figure 13 the dotted line represents what the patient perceives while the solid line indicates the reality of the relationship.

Figure 13.   A Barrier to Prayer

A common problem for most seriously ill patients is an overwhelming sense of isolation. Whether or not a seriously ill person has a strong support system, he or she often feels alone and cut off from human relationships. A thirty-three-year-old woman with a brain tumor describes her sense of isolation:

It is difficult to express the deep inner cravings of my heart during these last few months. I longed night and day for someone to reach out to me with an understanding hand and heart. It was as if I had a huge gaping wound that was unable to be treated. The pain, the fear, the irritability, the turmoil pressed upon me daily. It seemed as though no one was near me, no one cared. I thought I would collapse for want of understanding. I felt that I must be the only person to have ever experienced such a need.

The fact that warm, loving friends and family surround the person does not always cut through that sense of isolation.

When a patient cannot perceive the love and concern of other people, whom he can see, his ability to sense God's presence and concern is even further impaired. Often persons who have had stronger than usual faith will undergo the most distressing difficulties in their ability to pray. The woman with the brain tumor was a missionary, yet she concluded, "I needed someone to say in words the things I was unable to say to God." She was comforted because others were praying for her.

Our prayers for our patients are important, not only for the comfort the patients may receive, but because God hears our prayers and answers. Christian nurses have a responsibility to pray for their patients. However, praying *with* patients has some additional advantages. Jesus instructed the disciples, "If two of you agree on earth about anything they ask, it will be done for them by my Father in heaven" (Mt. 18:19). Praying together is important to God. Praying together is also important to the patient. When we say, "I'll pray for you," without finding out what the patient wants us to pray for, we may be of some comfort, but we offer only minimal support. The patient never knows what we will pray, nor does he or she have the assurance that we really did pray. As seen in Figure 14 the patient perceives no relationship with God or with the nurse (the dotted lines) despite the reality of our and the patient's relationships with God (the solid lines).

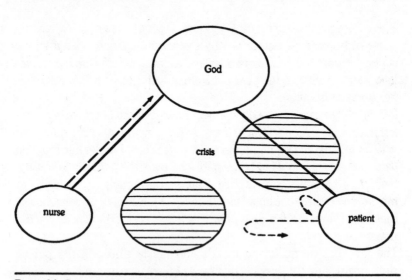

Figure 14. Failure to Meet a Spiritual Need through Prayer

When we pray with a patient at the bedside, the patient is assured of our awareness of and concern for his needs because he has heard us express those needs to God. The patient's relationship to God may be facilitated as he temporarily channels his prayer through us. We may also break through the barrier the patient feels interpersonally, as seen in Figure 15.

Shared prayer has some unique interpersonal side effects: it can be one of the deepest forms of human communication. Daniel DeArment claims that shared prayer allows "intimacy without exposure."[2] When we pray with a patient, expressing to God what the patient has told us both verbally and nonverbally, we break through the patient's isolation without directly confronting him with what we have observed but he has not said. For instance, a patient may deny he is fearful of surgery, but his affect betrays him. To confront that patient directly with, "You *are* afraid; I can tell," would probably send his defenses up further. But to pray with him, "Lord, comfort John tonight; calm his fears," might free him to talk about the fear he is experiencing.

The question of meaning can be dealt with much more deeply in shared prayer than in usual conversation. Travelbee asserts that one of

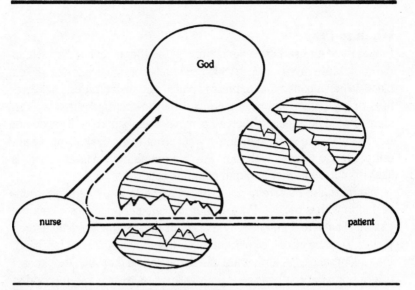

Figure 15. Meeting a Spiritual Need through Prayer

the key functions of a nurse is to help a patient find meaning in the experience of illness.[3] A relationship with God can supply meaning when human reason cannot satisfactorily explain the experience of illness. In praying with the patient we do more than assist the patient; we join him in his quest for meaning and go with him to the source of meaning.

When crisis has distorted a patient's view of God, we may be able to reveal a healthy concept of God to him or her through shared prayer. The patient may feel that God is far away and does not hear. His perception of God's love and concern may be renewed as we pray personally and confidently.

Perhaps the most significant factor in the use of prayer as a nursing resource is the work of the Holy Spirit. His activity within us cannot be explained scientifically, but it is a reality. Romans 8:26 states, "Likewise the Spirit helps us in our weakness; for we do not know how to pray as we ought, but the Spirit himself intercedes for us with sighs too deep for words." The observable interpersonal dynamics—the sense of intimacy and unity—which result from shared prayer do not attest to a psychological gimmick. They demonstrate the power of a personal God at work in his creatures.

When to Pray

Prayer must be used in conjunction with the therapeutic use of self, in the context of a relationship in which adequate communication has taken place. When a patient has expressed pain, fear, anxiety, stress, helplessness or joy (either verbally or nonverbally) to the extent that we can identify what he is feeling, then we can pray therapeutically. If we do not have a fairly clear understanding of what is bothering the patient, we are not yet ready to pray with him. Praying prematurely with a patient is likely to cut off further in-depth communication.

We must also be careful not to use prayer as a way of ending a conversation with a patient. Prayer often triggers deep feelings within the patient. The verbal interaction between us and the patient after shared prayer may be more significant than the conversation beforehand. DeArment states, "A further test of a dynamic and thoroughly legitimate use of prayer at the bedside is your willingness to stay and respond to the feelings and words of the patients which the prayer has touched."[4]

In situations where anxiety is characteristically higher than usual we should be alert to the patient's spiritual needs. Prayer can be especially helpful to the anxious patient preoperatively, before major tests, after admission to an unfamiliar environment or upon application of potentially frightening equipment (for example, respirators, electrodes, monitors).

Patients who give strong cues that their faith is important to them by verbal references, religious reading material and private devotions may greatly appreciate a nurse who offers to pray with them. Such patients may feel alienated from their faith community and find comfort in the nurse's offer of fellowship.

A basic guideline to determine the appropriateness of prayer in a given situation is to ask ourselves, "Whose need am I meeting—my own or the patient's?" If it is our own need that compels us to pray, then we would do better to pray privately or with a friend rather than to use the patient to meet our need.

Once we have determined we are meeting the patient's need by offering to pray with him, we have reached the planning stage of the nursing process. Prayer as a nursing measure must be couched in the context of the nursing process. It must be an appropriate response to a responsible assessment of the patient's needs.

How to Pray

When we pray with a patient, we express to God what the patient would pray if he were able. The most helpful prayer is usually a short, simple statement to God of the patient's hopes, fears and needs, and a recognition of God's ability to meet the patient in his situation.

Case 20. Rose Wade, age thirty-five, was admitted with a gunshot wound of the nose and mouth inflicted by her husband during an argument. Her condition was stable. She was alert, but she could not talk because of the pain and swelling of her tongue. She appeared frightened and uncomfortable. After orienting her to her surroundings, the nurse brought her a pencil and pad of paper and asked her to write down any questions or needs she might have. Rose wrote, "Where are my babies? What did they do with my husband? How long do I have to stay here?" The nurse promised to try to find the answers to Rose's questions and went out to the desk to make the necessary phone calls.

The babies were located at a neighbor's house. The nurse then called the neighbor from Rose's bedside phone in order to be able to reassure Rose that they were fine. Her husband was in jail. Rose's physician could give no estimate of the length of her stay. It would depend on her progress. After receiving the information she had requested, Rose seemed less distressed but still quite anxious. She wrote, "I love my husband. It was an *accident*. I don't want them to lock him up!" Then she lay back with a hopeless look. The nurse asked, "Rose, would you like me to pray with you?" Rose looked relieved and nodded.

The nurse prayed, "Father, thank you that you know what's going on in all this confusion. Thank you that Rose's babies are being well taken care of. We pray that you would be with her husband in jail and ask that he would be treated fairly. Give him peace, Lord. Help him to know that Rose loves him and you love him. Give strength and healing to Rose now, so she can go home again soon. She's frightened right now, please comfort her. In Jesus' name. Amen." ∎

In the prayer the nurse mentioned the problems Rose had brought up—her babies, her husband and her length of stay. The nurse, sensitive to Rose's nonverbal communication, also prayed that Rose's husband would know Rose loved him. At that point in the prayer Rose began to weep, indicating that a deep feeling had been touched. The nurse also recognized Rose's fright in the prayer, although they had not discussed it directly. The nurse prayed what Rose would have prayed, had she been able.

If we are to pray as the patient would pray, we need to consider the religious background of the patient, including the type of prayers which have been meaningful to him in the past. Most patients appreciate the simple, informal expression of their needs to God, but many persons have been accustomed to formal, written prayers. Some people may even feel that spontaneous prayers are disrespectful to God and may prefer a selected prayer from a prayer book. The Lord's Prayer is familiar and meaningful to most Christians. Often senile or semicomatose patients will be able to pray the Lord's Prayer with a nurse even when they are unable to respond to other verbal stimuli. Roman Catholic patients may appreciate having a nurse of the same faith who is willing to pray the rosary with them.

At times we may feel unable to pray what a patient would like us to pray.

Case 21. Mrs. Stevens, age sixty-nine, was lying in bed moaning and grasping the stump of her leg. A nurse passed her doorway. Mrs. Stevens called out, "Nurse, nurse, please pray for me." The nurse entered the room and sat down. "What do you want me to pray for?" "Pray that my leg would grow back," Mrs. Stevens replied.

(What could the nurse say to Mrs. Stevens?

1. If the nurse prayed for Mrs. Stevens as she requested, the nurse would reinforce Mrs. Stevens' unrealistic expectations. Prayer would be reduced to magic. God would be seen as a genie who grants wishes. If Mrs. Stevens' leg did not grow back, she might be convinced that God had failed her and did not really care about her.

2. The nurse could say, "Mrs. Stevens, I can't do that! Both you and I know that your leg will not grow back." Although this approach would be reality based, it would be treating Mrs. Stevens in a condescending manner. She might stop communicating her needs altogether. Mrs. Stevens needs love and support from the nurse and from God, not criticism.

3. A more constructive response would be, "It must really hurt to lose a leg." The nurse would then be giving Mrs. Stevens an opening to talk

about the loss she is experiencing and offering an empathetic ear. After Mrs. Stevens has had the opportunity to express her concerns related to the loss of the leg, the nurse will be able to pray more specifically for Mrs. Stevens' needs. How then does a nurse turn a patient's magical expectations into an appropriate and compassionate prayer?)

In talking with Mrs. Stevens the nurse found she was afraid of becoming dependent on her children or being forced to go to a nursing home. Her progress in physical therapy had been slow. She lived alone and was not at all sure she would be able to care for herself. She was also experiencing phantom pains in her amputated leg which made her fear she was losing her mind. After talking with Mrs. Stevens a few minutes, the nurse asked, "Why don't we pray about the things we've been talking about?" Mrs. Stevens agreed and the nurse prayed: "Heavenly Father, thank you that you know Mrs. Stevens and love her very much. Thank you too that you know her needs. Father, you know how frightened she is right now. Her life seems to be changing so much all at once and there are so many unknowns. Father, give her courage and strength. Help her in physical therapy and give her confidence as she learns to walk with the artificial leg. Lord, we know that you are in control of Mrs. Stevens' future and you will provide for her as she leaves the hospital. Give her your peace now. Ease her pain and let her get some good rest tonight. Thank you for being with her. In Jesus' name. Amen."■

The nurse's prayer communicated that God loves Mrs. Stevens, he knows her needs and he is with her. It was specifically related to the actual needs expressed by the patient, but it did not raise unrealistic expectations.

Prayer is not magic. Prayer is communication in a relationship between God and us. We cannot manipulate God by demanding unrealistic answers. Mrs. Stevens' request was clearly a desire for a magical act on God's part.

Nurses are often confronted with requests which may not be asking for something overtly magical but which may raise questions. At what point does it become inappropriate to ask God for results? How specific can we be with our requests? Can we ever pray for healing for a patient? If so, when?

Perhaps the most helpful guidelines on how to pray come from a clear understanding of the nature of God's relationship to us. Communicating with our heavenly Father is not unlike talking with our earthly parents in many respects. Because we know our parents well, we soon learn to anticipate which requests will be granted and which ones will not. In a healthy parent-child relationship the child also knows his parents love him even if they do not allow him to do or have everything he wants. A child comes to his parents for other reasons than to make requests. He expresses his thoughts and feelings to his parents. He shares his activities and his dreams. He communicates love and appreciation. He learns to say thank you.

Prayer involves the same type of interaction as child-parent communication. God as heavenly Father is a much more mature view of God than God as genie. When we with our patients approach God as our Father, we are sharing a mature concept of God with them.

The Bible presents God as a loving Father who gives "good things to those who ask him" (Mt. 7:11). Included in those good things is healing. Healing in a biblical sense, however, is more inclusive than mere physical healing. Health and salvation are closely related in Scripture. The Hebrew word for salvation may also be translated "saving health." God is concerned about the whole person. We are told in the Scriptures to pray for healing (for example, Jas. 5:13-15). Physical healing may result from our prayers,[5] but not necessarily.[6] God's central concern is that each person live in vital relationship to him.

When we pray with a patient, we bring comfort and encouragement through facilitating the patient's relationship with God. We can also facilitate that relationship by being alert to patients who may desire a period of privacy for personal devotions or an undisturbed visit from a pastor. Prayer is a vital link with God. We help patients experience God's meaning and purpose, love, and forgiveness as we pray with them at the bedside.

Chapter 7
The Use
of Scripture

For whatever was written in former days
was written for our instruction, that by
steadfastness and by the encouragement of the
scriptures we might have hope.
Romans 15:4

The Old and New Testaments are God's personal communication to us. The Bible was written by individuals inspired by the Holy Spirit.[1] Its primary purpose is to enable people to establish a dynamic, personal relationship with God through Jesus Christ and to teach people how to maintain harmonious relationships with God, themselves and others.[2]

Illness is an unsteady state which can cause physical, psychosocial and spiritual disharmony or disequilibrium. It can create a very real need for stability—for some integrating force that will hold the pieces together of a life that may seem fragmentized and devoid of meaning and purpose, love or forgiveness.

Case 22. Mrs. McCauley had been a Sunday-school teacher for forty years before a cardiovascular accident left her severely affected and unable to walk. A public health nurse visited her weekly. One day after the nurse completed her care and was preparing to leave, Mrs. McCauley asked her, "Would you please read me a psalm? I have trouble focusing my eyes and miss being able to read the Bible."

The nurse was familiar with the Psalms and chose one she felt Mrs. McCauley would appreciate. She read Psalm 71. Mrs. McCauley sat up with a jolt when the nurse came to verses 17 and 18:

O God, from my youth thou hast taught me,
  and I still proclaim thy wondrous deeds.
So even to old age and gray hairs,
  O God, do not forsake me,
till I proclaim thy might
  to all the generations to come.

"I've been so depressed lately," Mrs. McCauley told the nurse when she had finished reading. "I thought God was through with me on this earth. But according to the psalm, he's not! He's still got work for me to do!" ■

Scripture, when used appropriately with patients, can be like a light at the end of a long, dark tunnel. It can provide the glimmer of something better. Paul stated in Romans 15:4, "For whatever was written in former days was written for our instruction, that by steadfastness and by the encouragement of the scriptures we might have hope."

The Bible can provide hope in crisis and meet spiritual needs because it focuses our attention on a stable, dependable God who has chosen to communicate his character and will to people like Mrs. McCauley who need to know that God cares about them. It tells us that God the Father is in complete control of the world and that he gives meaning and purpose to all of life, including suffering, old age and death.[3] God the Son, Jesus Christ, is called "Savior" in Scripture; he is able to meet our need for forgiveness.[4] Jesus is also called a shepherd who meets our need for love and relatedness.[5]

The Scriptures speak of a variety of gifts given by God to meet the needs of people in the church. Many of these gifts are related to the use of Scripture. Some people are to be preachers, others teachers and interpreters. They are to instruct people in the various doctrines of the Christian faith and reprove and correct when necessary.[6] The role of the nurse in using Scripture with patients seems to fall into the category of a helper or comforter, who brings a word of encouragement to someone who is suffering.

This hope-giving aspect of Scripture and the role and responsibility of a comforter is described in Isaiah 50:4: "The Lord GOD has given me the tongue of those who are taught, that I may know how to sustain with a word him that is weary. Morning by morning he wakens, he wakens my ear to hear as those who are taught."

One of the nurse's personal resources is a knowledge of Scripture. The public health nurse who visited Mrs. McCauley was able to be a comforter and use the Scripture therapeutically because of her familiarity with the content of the Psalms. Nurses who desire to "sustain with a word" a weary patient will be most effective if they are able to share from their own relationship with God what Scripture has been meaningful to them and is relevant to the needs their patient may be expressing.

Paul Tournier, a Swiss physician who has written numerous books on the relationship between medicine and religion, has devoted one book to the relationship between medicine and the Bible. He encourages doctors to study the Bible with their profession in mind, always asking the question, What does the Bible have to say about the patient as a person, life and death, disease and sin, and relationships with patients?[7] Nurses need to ask similar questions. What does the Bible have to say to a patient who is facing surgery, approaching death or suffering from a chronic illness? What does the Bible have to teach us about meaning and purpose, love and relatedness, and forgiveness? Our answers to these questions will help us determine the appropriate use of Scripture with patients in need of a word of comfort.

When to Use Scripture

We are most likely to be helpful to persons in crisis if we use an economy of words. We usually talk far too much. We should spend more time listening. Joseph Bayly, in his book *The View from a Hearse*, describes his feelings after the death of a son:

I was sitting, torn by grief. Someone came and talked to me of God's dealings, of why it happened, of hope beyond the grave. He talked constantly, he said things I knew were true.

I was unmoved, except to wish he'd go away. He finally did.

Another came and sat beside me. He didn't talk. He didn't ask leading questions. He just sat beside me for an hour and more, listened when I said something, answered briefly, prayed simply, left.

I was moved. I was comforted. I hated to see him go.[8]

One principle that governs the use of Scripture with patients is the principle of appropriate timing. Proverbs says singing songs to a heavy heart is like taking off a person's coat on a cold day or pouring vinegar on a wound (25:20). There is nothing inherently wrong with singing songs, but if they are sung at an inappropriate time, they will fall on deaf ears. The same is true of the use of Scripture. Right answers about God given at the wrong moment are of little therapeutic value. The answers fail to comfort and in fact they may do a person more harm than good.

The first man who visited Joseph Bayly was undoubtedly filled with good intentions and right thoughts about God and the afterlife. But he failed to consider the needs of the mourning father, who simply wanted someone to sit with him, to listen and to enter into his personal experience of grief.

The premature use of Scripture can be compared to putting salve on a festering wound that first needs a good débridement. A person who is suffering or grieving may initially need to talk about his situation—to express his feelings, vent his anger, cry, "be real" with another person who can accept him nonjudgmentally.

A visiting nurse describes her own crisis in dealing with the chronic illness of friends and the inappropriate and therapeutic use of Scripture:

November: It was my first V.N.A. visit to Mrs. Sloan. Eight years ago she'd had a radical mastectomy. Now she was in severe pain with many open lesions on her chest. She was calling out to God and we began to talk about spiritual things. I prayed with her before I left that day and God answered miraculously in giving her relief from pain. During the succeeding months we prayed for each other often. God had used me to encourage her and show His love for her.

March: I was angry at God! Several dear friends were suffering with chronic diseases. One who had surgery had many complications and was basically confined to her bed for months. There seemed to be no progress, only decline. I found it hard to pray. I'd been praying specifically— for sleep, for pain relief, but I wasn't seeing answers. I felt helpless and hopeless!

April: This weekend at work, I was called to reopen a case. It was Mrs. Sloan. She was now in the terminal stages of cancer. She wanted to die. Friends were praying that God would take her home soon. "I've prayed for death, but God must want me to stay around a little longer for some reason. He has given me the twenty-third Psalm." She repeated it twice while I was there that day and kept praising God and expressing her anticipation of soon seeing Jesus.

She did not know it but she was now meeting her nurse's need. I needed to see hope in an unimproving situation. God allowed me to see it in Mrs. Sloan. It gave me encouragement and hope which a well person could never have given me.

May: What have I learned these past few months? I've learned that

God is the answer. But I've also learned to consider whether now is the appropriate time to talk about this fact.

When I was struggling with my feelings and reactions to the suffering of my friends, I was not comforted by Christians who told me, "God has things in control—things will work out all right" and then read Scripture. Instead I became angry. I felt it was easy for them to say all that when they were on a mountain top or plateau experience with God, but I was in a valley seeing no change or hope for change. I needed someone who would accept my anger and irritability and listen without saying much. Sometimes I needed to cry and just have someone touch me or hold me.

Having the right answer or quoting Scripture too quickly may put up a barrier which prevents an individual from being real. This increases loneliness. One friend listened, shared what had helped her in a similar situation, communicated caring and then shared some Scripture and prayed with me. This was helpful because I felt her love and care for me and for the first time in a long time, I felt the presence of God. Then the Scriptures were more meaningful and provided comfort because He loved me through a friend.

God has taught me much this year. I believe He has provided these learning experiences so that I could more fully understand what my patients are going through in order to support, comfort and encourage them. [9]

Applying Bible passages too quickly can create unnecessary barriers to communication. The patient may become angry at the nurse. This can inhibit further expression of needs. A nurse who uses Scripture prematurely may also communicate an impersonal God who has a pat answer to every question but refuses to concern himself with the real feelings and frustrations of suffering human beings who need compassionate understanding. For a patient who has little knowledge of the Bible and may be questioning God's existence and involvement in his life, pat answers from the Scriptures can serve to alienate him further from God. They can also reinforce the idea that the Bible is merely a book of rules and regulations—a book of correction rather than a book of comfort.

The sharing of Scripture, like shared prayer, should bring a patient and nurse closer together, and open the door for further communication.

The use of Scripture should also bring a person closer to God. Nurses who are willing first to listen and then to empathize with a patient, to feel his pain and loss, to weep with him, sit with him and *then* to consider Scripture passages which have been helpful in their own experience should be able to use Scripture therapeutically. Nurses who are patient enough to listen to a suffering person's concerns and simply comfort him on a human level with their presence can help communicate the presence of a personal God. *A word of comfort should be given in the context of a meaningful personal relationship.*

We noted that one basic question we can use to determine the appropriate use of prayer with patients is, "Whose need am I meeting?" This question can help us identify our *motivation* for using Scripture with a patient. Are we meeting our patient's need for spiritual comfort and support or our own need to give spiritual advice and counsel?

The book of Job gives a graphic illustration of the improperly motivated and compulsive use of Scripture. Job has three friends who come to comfort him in his crisis. Their visit soon turns into a visit of affliction. They bombard Job with countless facts about God in an attempt to discover the cause and cure for Job's sufferings. They are motivated by their preconceived ideas about the way God deals with human beings. William Hulme says they are also driven by their need to "defend the ways of God" and by a compulsion to turn Job's negative thoughts about God into a positive conversation that would relieve their own anxieties.[10] Job verbally lashes out at them, accusing them of being miserable comforters and worthless physicians who are failing to meet his felt needs for love and understanding (Job 13:4; 16:2).

Nurses who use Scripture compulsively may do so for reasons similar to the motivations of Job's friends. These reasons are related to the barriers we discussed earlier—word meanings, preconceptions, anxiety, defenses, purposes and values. For example, nurses who are aware that one of God's purposes is to draw people into a saving relationship with himself through faith in Jesus Christ may assume the role of an evangelist with every patient they believe does not have a personal and dynamic relationship with God. They may feel if they neglect to witness verbally for Christ by sharing what it means to become a Christian, and do not use Scripture related to this theme, they will have somehow failed

God. They can be easily motivated by guilt. If they neglect to share their faith, their anxiety level may increase and prevent them from accurately assessing other needs their patient may be expressing. If they do share their beliefs and the patient becomes defensive, they may react by becoming defensive themselves and beginning a religious argument that may include proof-texts. This may only serve to drive the patient further from God. All this does not mean that nurses should never share with a patient how to establish a relationship with God. It does mean that sharing must be properly motivated and in response to an expressed need.

How to Use Scripture

It is important to know when to use prayer and Scripture. The content of the prayers we pray and the Scripture we share is also important. A patient's needs are our primary guide for determining the appropriate Scripture passage to use. A patient may request a passage of Scripture that has been meaningful in the past.

Case 23. Mrs. Wilson was an elderly resident of a nursing home who suffered from headaches and dizzy spells. She spent her days sitting alone on the third floor solarium by her room. She had been in the home for eight years and had few visitors. One day Mrs. Wilson asked a nurse to read the Bible to her. She had shared previously with the nurse about the importance of church to her in the past and her close relationship with the Lord. The nurse had prayed with Mrs. Wilson about her physical concerns.

The nurse noted that Mrs. Wilson seemed more depressed than usual and was verbalizing feelings of loneliness. The nurse asked Mrs. Wilson if she had a favorite passage of Scripture. Mrs. Wilson requested Psalm 25. The nurse read the entire psalm and then reread verses 14-18:

The friendship of the LORD is for those who fear him,
and he makes known to them his covenant.
My eyes are ever toward the LORD,
for he will pluck my feet out of the net.
Turn thou to me, and be gracious to me;
for I am lonely and afflicted.
Relieve the troubles of my heart,
and bring me out of my distresses.

Consider my affliction and my trouble,
  and forgive all my sins.

After reading these verses the nurse spent a few minutes talking with Mrs. Wilson about the friendship of the Lord. Mrs. Wilson then shared with the nurse how thankful she was for God's faithfulness to her and the hope he now gave her in sending her a special friend like the nurse to read his Word to her.■

The use of Scripture with Mrs. Wilson opened up the door for further communication in a brief but meaningful interaction. This also gave Mrs. Wilson an opportunity to reflect on what God meant to her and to recognize his faithfulness to her.

The following example illustrates a situation when a patient did not request Scripture but appreciated a nurse's use of it:

Case 24.   The nurse entered the room. Mrs. Carlson, a forty-eight-year-old diabetic, was fingering her bed linen and trying hard not to cry.

"What's wrong, Mrs. Carlson?" the nurse asked.

"Nothing," Mrs. Carlson replied curtly. "Leave me alone!"

The nurse left the room but returned an hour later.

"I'm sorry for being so rude to you," Mrs. Carlson began. "It's just that sometimes it's so hard to be cheerful. I try to put up a front. My husband expects it, you know. So do my children. We've brought them up to believe in God and to trust him in all things. I know it's wrong to be angry. I promise I won't yell at you again."

(The nurse in this situation could have done one of several things:

1. The nurse could have passed off Mrs. Carlson's final comment with a shrug and said something like, "That's all right, Mrs. Carlson. We all have our bad days. Forget it." While there would have been some merit in the nurse's not taking Mrs. Carlson's curtness personally, passing off this comment as something that was not in the least bothersome may have also communicated to Mrs. Carlson that her feelings did not matter to the nurse either. Or she may have felt they were unacceptable. This may have erected a further barrier to communication.

2. The nurse could have said, "Yes, Mrs. Carlson, you are right. The Bible does say in Romans 8:28 that all things work together for good to those who love God. He will take care of our problems if we just trust him." A statement like this would have denied Mrs. Carlson's under-

lying feelings of anger and could have compounded the guilt she already felt at being angry with God.

3. What the nurse did was to assess the situation. Mrs. Carlson had mentioned that God was important to her and to others in her family. She also gave some clues about her relationship with God and her concept of God. She believed God could not, or would not, accept anger. She felt anger was a sin because it indicated lack of trust. The image of herself as a person who trusted God was being attacked by her inability to maintain her composure in a difficult situation.)

The nurse offered to talk with Mrs. Carlson and explored her feelings in a nonthreatening and empathetic way. The nurse began by telling Mrs. Carlson it was all right for her to be angry: "If I were in your situation, I'd be angry too. Maybe it would help to talk about it."

Mrs. Carlson began to weep and share frustrations that were related to her uncontrolled diabetes and her spiritual struggles. God seemed very remote and unconcerned. Mrs. Carlson felt she had alienated God by her lack of trust and feelings of anger. She was afraid of doing the same thing to her husband and children, but it was becoming increasingly difficult to remain cheerful when they came to visit.

The nurse listened and then told Mrs. Carlson about a time of feeling anger toward God in a difficult situation. When the nurse asked Mrs. Carlson for permission to share some Scripture verses that had been helpful at that time, Mrs. Carlson agreed. The nurse turned to Psalm 13 and read:

How long, O LORD? Wilt thou forget me for ever?
How long wilt thou hide thy face from me?
How long must I bear pain in my soul,
 and have sorrow in my heart all the day?
How long shall my enemy be exalted over me?
Consider and answer me, O LORD my God;
 lighten my eyes, lest I sleep the sleep of death;
lest my enemy say, "I have prevailed over him";
 lest my foes rejoice because I am shaken.
But I have trusted in thy steadfast love;
 my heart shall rejoice in thy salvation.
I will sing to the LORD,
 because he has dealt bountifully with me. (Ps. 13:1-6)

"That psalm helped me," said the nurse, "because it made me realize that people in the Bible became angry and frustrated, and were able to be honest with God about their feelings. I realized I could talk to God and give him my unacceptable feelings and he wouldn't desert me." Mrs. Carlson then began to express more of her angry feelings to the nurse and asked to see the hospital chaplain. She also asked the nurse to pray for her to be more honest in expressing her real feelings to her husband when he visited and to be honest and open with God. ■

Psalm 13 could be considered an "identification passage." It helped Mrs. Carlson realize she was neither alone in her struggles nor the first person to be angry with God. The Psalms are a rich source of identification passages for feelings ranging from anxiety, anger, depression and guilt to joy, elation, praise and thanksgiving. Used appropriately, they can be a source of comfort and can help a patient identify and accept his own feelings.

Identification passages are also an aid to prayer. A patient who is having difficulty communicating his feelings and thoughts to God may be able to express them through the words of a psalm. For example, a patient who is in need of forgiveness and desires to confess his sin could find help in Psalm 51.

Have mercy on me, O God, according to thy steadfast love;
   according to thy abundant mercy blot out my transgressions.
Wash me thoroughly from my iniquity,
   and cleanse me from my sin! (Ps. 51:1-2)

In the remaining verses of the psalm, the psalmist acknowledges his guilt more specifically, confesses his sin and asks God to restore to him the joy of his salvation.

A patient who has been depressed due to a serious illness and is now on the road to recovery might be able to see his or her own situation mirrored in the opening verses of Psalm 40:

I waited patiently for the LORD;
   he inclined to me and heard my cry.
He drew me up from the desolate pit,
   out of the miry bog,
and set my feet upon a rock,
   making my steps secure.

He put a new song in my mouth,
 a song of praise to our God. (Ps. 40:1-3)
Case 25. Mrs. Hutchins was a forty-five-year-old woman who had
been admitted for a breast biopsy. Much to her surprise and relief, the
tumor was benign. After the biopsy Mrs. Hutchins seemed to be bubbling
over with joy. "I just want to thank the Lord!" she exclaimed to a nurse,
clapping her hands.■

Psalm 92 was an appropriate psalm of thanksgiving for Mrs. Hutchins:

It is good to give thanks to the LORD,
 to sing praises to thy name, O Most High;
to declare thy steadfast love in the morning,
 and thy faithfulness by night,
to the music of the lute and the harp,
 to the melody of the lyre.
For thou, O LORD, hast made me glad by thy work;
 at the works of thy hands I sing for joy. (Ps. 92:1-4)

The feelings expressed by patients can help us know how to use
certain identification passages. Other passages of Scripture can be applied
to specific nursing situations.[11]

A patient who is facing surgery or diagnostic procedures is confronted
by a host of fears and anxieties. Scripture passages that focus on God's
control of every situation may be of help to quiet such a patient's
heart and bring a sense of peace. Psalm 139 is a reminder that God
made us, knows our thoughts and feelings, and is present with us in all
situations. Psalm 121 describes the Lord as an ever-watchful keeper or
guardian:

I lift up my eyes to the hills.
 From whence does my help come?
My help comes from the LORD,
 who made heaven and earth.

He will not let your foot be moved,
 he who keeps you will not slumber.
Behold, he who keeps Israel
 will neither slumber nor sleep.

The LORD is your keeper;
    the LORD is your shade
    on your right hand.
The sun shall not smite you by day,
    nor the moon by night.

The LORD will keep you from all evil;
    he will keep your life.
The LORD will keep
    your going out and your coming in
    from this time forth and for evermore.

Two New Testament passages from Philippians and 1 Peter recognize anxiety as a legitimate feeling and encourage people to cast their anxiety on the Lord, who gives peace and cares for us. These verses, coupled with Romans 8:38-39, could give added courage to a person who is fearful and anxious and in need of the reassurance of God's presence and love.

Rejoice in the Lord always; again I will say, Rejoice. Let all men know your forbearance. The Lord is at hand. Have no anxiety about anything, but in everything by prayer and supplication with thanksgiving let your requests be made known to God. And the peace of God, which passes all understanding, will keep your hearts and minds in Christ Jesus. (Phil. 4:4-7)

Cast all your anxieties on him, for he cares about you. (1 Pet. 5:7)

For I am sure that neither death, nor life, nor angels, nor principalities, nor things present, nor things to come, nor powers, nor height, nor depth, nor anything else in all creation, will be able to separate us from the love of God in Christ Jesus our Lord. (Rom. 8:38-39)

A patient who is approaching death may also be beset by many fears. John 14:1-7 is a particularly helpful passage. It begins by focusing on the fears of Jesus' disciples, whose hearts were troubled with the thought of Jesus' coming death. They may also have feared their own death. The fear of the unknown which often accompanies the last stages of life was also recognized by Jesus, who described heaven in terms the disciples could relate to. For a person who has never established a personal relationship with God through faith in Christ, or is lacking assurance of eternal life, this passage also presents clearly the means of establishing that relationship:

"Let not your hearts be troubled; believe in God, believe also in me. In my Father's house are many rooms; if it were not so, would I have told you that I go to prepare a place for you? And when I go and prepare a place for you, I will come again and will take you to myself, that where I am you may be also. And you know the way where I am going." Thomas said to him, "Lord, we do not know where you are going; how can we know the way?" Jesus said to him, "I am the way, and the truth, and the life; no one comes to the Father, but by me. If you had known me, you would have known my Father also; henceforth you know him and have seen him." (Jn. 14:1-7)

1 Corinthians 15 can provide comfort for a patient who has questions about the reality and nature of the resurrection body. Psalm 23 is the traditional psalm of comfort. It describes God as a tender shepherd who leads his people through the valley of the shadow of death.

The need for forgiveness can be experienced by a patient at any time. The fear of death may cause this need to be more evident. The passages below speak of God's mercy and his desire to forgive and of our need to confess our sin and receive forgiveness through Jesus Christ.

"Come now, let us reason together, says the LORD:
though your sins are like scarlet,
  they shall be as white as snow;
though they are red like crimson,
  they shall become like wool." (Is. 1:18)

But he was wounded for our transgressions,
  he was bruised for our iniquities;
upon him was the chastisement that made us whole,
  and with his stripes we are healed.
All we like sheep have gone astray;
  we have turned every one to his own way;
and the LORD has laid on him
  the iniquity of us all. (Is. 53:5-6)

Since then we have a great high priest who has passed through the heav-

ens, Jesus, the Son of God, let us hold fast our confession. For we have not
a high priest who is unable to sympathize with our weaknesses, but one
who in every respect has been tempted as we are, yet without sin. Let us
then with confidence draw near to the throne of grace, that we may
receive mercy and find grace to help in time of need. (Heb. 4:14-16)

If we confess our sins, he is faithful and just, and will forgive our sins and
cleanse us from all unrighteousness. (1 Jn. 1:9)

A patient who is suffering from a chronic illness may be experiencing
feelings of despair, frustration and loneliness. A nurse should be careful
not to deny the patient's feelings by quoting Scripture prematurely, but
Scripture that focuses on God's purposes for suffering may be of help.
2 Corinthians 1:3-11 describes God as a God of all comfort who enables
us to endure suffering and gives us the strength to turn our suffering into
help for others. For some patients this "help for others" may take the
form of intercessory prayer.

Isaiah 43 can also provide the reassurance that the Lord is with us in
crisis, especially verse 2:
When you pass through the waters I will be with you;
    and through the rivers, they shall not overwhelm you;
when you walk through fire you shall not be burned,
    and the flame shall not consume you. (Is. 43:2)

A patient who may be able to see only his own suffering and distress
might be helped by focusing his attention on the sufferings of Christ.
Isaiah 53 could be used in conjunction with Romans 5:1-5, which encourages us to rejoice in our sufferings because they produce endurance,
character and the hope of sharing the glory of God.

For the elderly, crisis can create a longing for the old and the familiar.
Passages of Scripture that the patient is well acquainted with are usually
welcomed and can help restore a sense of stability.

Case 26. One nurse discovered that Mr. Foster, an elderly man on
the unit, always repeated the twenty-third Psalm with his wife at bedtime.
His wife, though, was unable to visit regularly. So the nurse wrote on
the evening medication card: "HS Medication: Read 23rd Psalm from
patient's Bible." ■

The nurses were able to bring comfort to Mr. Foster by assisting him in continuing a long-established practice.

A nurse should be sensitive in choosing a translation if a patient does not have a Bible at the bedside.

Case 27. Anne, a registered nurse, was visiting her mother in the intensive care unit. Mrs. Brown was recovering from an acute myocardial infarction. She had a deep love for the Lord and for the Scriptures and seemed alert and cheerful.

"Mom," Anne asked, "would you like me to read the Scriptures?"

"Of course," her mother replied.

Anne had brought along her own Bible, a modern translation and proceeded to read Romans 8. After reading she looked up, expecting to dialog with her mother.

Mrs. Brown looked exasperated. "That was not the King James Version, was it daughter? That, of course, is the original." ■

All eighty-seven-year-old mothers may not be as fond of the King's English as was Mrs. Brown, but for many people who have been raised on one particular translation of the Bible, all others may have a ring of unreality.

Joni Eareckson, a young quadriplegic struggling to find meaning in life after a diving accident, wrote a book based on her experiences. She describes the importance of Scripture and the value of a particular translation that was shared by a friend: "Dick came by the hospital later. Quietly I lay there listening to the comforting words of Scripture he read to me from a J. B. Phillips New Testament paraphrase. Many of the verses were alive with contemporary meaning." After reading the passage and praying, Joni began to see more positive aspects about her accident.[12]

There may be times when a patient wants to share Scripture with the nurse. A young woman with severe hip pain confided to her nurse one day when her visitors had left, "People keep telling me where to look in the Scriptures. I wish they'd just ask me what I was learning from my experience. God has been showing me all kinds of exciting things in his Word. I need to share them."

Bibles can be obtained for hospitals, nursing homes and other health-care facilities through the Gideons International. Arrangements should be made through the chaplain's department and must be made with the approval of the hospital administration. The Gideons distribute Bibles in both the King James Version and the Berkeley Translation. They also distribute the New Testament with Psalms and Proverbs in a large-print edition.

The American Bible Society usually does not distribute free Bibles to health-care facilities, but Bibles can be ordered from them at low cost. Translations available include the King James Version, the Revised Standard Version and the Today's English Version (Good News Bible). Bibles in Braille are also available as are the New Testament and various Old Testament books on cassette tapes. The Bible can also be obtained in many foreign languages. Scripture portions printed on colorful cards can be ordered for a minimal cost.

Local branches of both the Gideons and the American Bible Society are located in large metropolitan areas. The national addresses are:

The Gideons International
2900 Lebanon Road
Nashville, Tennessee 37214

The American Bible Society
P. O. Box 5656, Grand Central Station
New York, New York 10017

The Scriptures are God's personal communication to us. They are the truth of God expressed in words, applicable to people in crisis. They should not be used like a crude tool, but accurately and precisely, like a delicate surgical instrument.

The use of Scripture is a skill we can develop. We begin to develop the skill by gaining a personal knowledge of the Bible and an understanding of our own motivations. We also need to increase our awareness of the needs and feelings of patients in crisis situations.

Proverbs 12:25 says, "Anxiety in a man's heart weighs him down, but a good word makes him glad." A nurse who brings a good word of comfort from Scripture may help to decrease the anxiety that is so much a part of the experience of illness.

Chapter 8
Referral to the Clergy

In one way or another, whether the minister likes it or not, he or she is faced with the crises in parishioners' lives. Crisis ministry has been part of pastoral care throughout many centuries in which Christians have learned to expect their pastors to be with them at crucial times.
Howard W. Stone

The clergy are another major resource in spiritual care. The ministry of the clergy and the spiritual care given by nurses should complement one another. For nurses and the clergy to function together effectively, several conditions must exist. First, there must be the common goal of caring for the whole person. Second, there must be a clear distinction of roles. Third, there must be an open channel of communication.

Common Goals

Both nurses and the clergy must have a clear focus on the patient as a whole person who is in need of the maintenance or restoration of health. The concept of the clergy as members of the health-care team is not new. Until about 1850 health care was considered to be the role of the church.[1] Most hospitals were established and run by churches. Members of the clergy worked in close association with the health-care team and often controlled hospital boards.

Gradually, as medicine became more scientific, the patient was compartmentalized so that the physician assumed care of the body and the clergy, of the soul. The nurse was left somewhere in between but leaning heavily toward physical care. We have already discussed the reasons why a dualistic view of man is untenable (see chapter two). Since man cannot be neatly divided into body and soul, both nurses and the clergy care for the whole person. However, they do so from different perspectives.

Distinct Roles

Without a clear distinction of functions, confusion may result when two professionals attempt to work toward the same goal in caring for the same individual. A study of interdisciplinary teamwork in a hospital setting revealed that members of the health sciences tend to be very protective of their professional roles. The result of this protective attitude is a "territorial imperialism" which makes teamwork difficult.[2] Clinebell asserts that if effective teamwork is to occur it is of central importance that "mutual understanding and appreciation of each other's unique competencies, views, insights, and contributions to the helping-healing enterprise" be developed.[3]

Part of our difficulty in defining the role of nurses in spiritual care, as distinct from the role of the clergy, is that both roles are in transition. Both nurses and clergy may feel insecure about meeting the spiritual needs of the hospitalized patient.[4] As they both become more confident and aware of their separate contributions to spiritual care, they can begin to work together. Nurses are distinct from the clergy in four major areas: (1) availability, (2) involvement, (3) education and experience, and (4) context and authority.

Nurses are *available* to hospitalized patients at the press of a call-button. They are the most readily accessible persons to patients. But they are available to all patients for whom they are responsible, which may make them feel rushed and pressured when they answer a particular patient's call. The amount of time nurses are able to spend with one patient is often determined by variables beyond their control; for example, the number of patients for whom they are responsible, the nature of their conditions and the adequacy of staffing. The clergy are able to plan periods of time with patients during which they can concentrate their full attention on the one person they are visiting. Although the clergy are rarely present at the time of an acute crisis or increased stress, they can arrive later to provide extended pastoral care. Nurses have the responsibility to provide immediate spiritual support in crisis and stress situations.

The length of a nurse's *involvement* with a patient is usually short-term, limited to the period of hospitalization. A hospital chaplain has the same limitation. A patient's own pastor has usually known the patient prior to his illness and is aware of how he and his family were able to cope with past crises. A nurse knows only the information on the patient's chart and whatever else the patient or his family reveals about themselves. This may be an advantage for the nurse. Frequently, the patient may feel more comfortable expressing doubts, fears and weaknesses to someone he did not know when he was strong and self-sufficient. He does not have a previous image to maintain. The disadvantage is that the patient-nurse relationship ends at discharge. The patient's pastor can provide continuity of care when he leaves the hospital. This continuity is especially important if the patient is transferred to the unfamiliar surroundings of a nursing home or rehabilitation center. The pastor will usually be aware of the patient's family and community resources. This knowledge should enable him to deal more comprehensively with the person's spiritual needs.

Not only the length of involvement but the level of involvement differs for nurses and the clergy. Beland quotes a study of distance between people in interaction which labeled 0 to 1½ feet as the "intimate zone," 1½ to 4 feet as the "personal zone," 4 to 12 feet as the "social zone," and 12 to 25 feet as the "public zone." In the hospital setting, nurses spend more time than anyone else in the intimate zone, and patients believe it is appropriate for them to do so. The intimate contact not only serves to meet physical needs but also communicates the nurse's respect and compassion for the patient.[5]

Once the barrier of the intimate zone is broken by the nurse providing physical care, the transition may be made to spiritual care while remaining on the same level of intimacy. The clergy do not have the natural entrée to intimacy which physical care provides nurses. Guilt over infrequent church attendance, past behavior or doubts about God may cause a patient to construct further barriers to communication with a minister.

While both nurses and members of the clergy are concerned with the well-being of the whole person, they differ in *education and experience*. Nurses approach patients from the vantage point of nursing science and nursing care; pastors come from the perspective of theology and pastoral care. Nurses focus on health and illness; pastors focus on spiritual growth and development. A nurse's theological understanding may be limited to personal beliefs; pastors should be able to understand a patient's religious background and relate to him accordingly. For example, the problem of sin and the need for confession and forgiveness may often require a pastor who can enter into the patient's religious framework to deal adequately with them. Nurses understand the dynamics and characteristics of illness and its effect on a patient's mental and emotional functioning. Pastors usually have a limited understanding of the disease process. Illness and drug-related behavior may be confusing and disconcerting to them. For nurses, illness is usually the norm in their experience with patients. To pastors illness is a rude interruption in the healthy life of their parishioners.

Nurses and the clergy also have a different perception of their *context and authority*. The hospital, which is home turf to nurses, is often foreign soil to pastors. It may even appear as a hostile and dehumanizing environment. Consider a pastor who has known a parishioner as an active, healthy person in the context of his family and church community. He receives word that the parishioner has been hospitalized. When he enters the hospital room he sees a semiconscious, disfigured person attached to bottles and machines by tubes and wires. He will have to deal with his own feelings as well as those of the patient and his family. He may also have to support distraught friends in the congregation. A nurse may be more emotionally detached from the patient and thus freer to respond to his spiritual concerns.

When nurses intervene, they represent the hospital community. Their spiritual intervention can also be an exercise of what Martin Luther called "the priesthood of all believers" (that is, all Christians have the responsibility to encourage and support one another). The clergy are official representatives of the church. They are ordained by a religious body and given specific responsibilities for which they are held accountable. In most Christian denominations those responsibilities include "the ministry of teaching the Gospel and administering the sacraments."[6] The spiritual intervention of the clergy carries official status. To some patients it will be the *only* spiritual assistance that is acceptable to them. To many Christians the sacrament of Holy Communion, or the Lord's Supper, is an important channel of God's grace. It may be especially meaningful during illness. Unless a nurse is an ordained minister, that nurse cannot serve communion to patients but can offer to contact the appropriate member of the clergy.

Open Communication

The ministry of the clergy and the spiritual care of nurses should complement one another. Clear channels of communication between them will facilitate the optimum functioning of both. Distrust and lack of respect result if nurses and clergy are not in direct communication.

A pastor should introduce himself to the nurse and report which patient he will be visiting. The nurse can return that courtesy by ensuring uninterrupted privacy for the visit. The nurse should also inform him of any spiritual needs the patient has expressed and any spiritual intervention taken by the nursing personnel. If a visiting pastor does not introduce himself, the nurse should take the initiative to make the introductions and make the pastor feel welcome.

Other helpful information nurses can communicate to the clergy includes insight into a patient's progress or condition, and an explanation of unusual behavior—labile emotions, drowsiness, confusion, slurred speech—especially if it is drug- or disease-related. It is also helpful to explain if a patient can hear but cannot respond appropriately.

Occasionally, a nurse may feel a particular pastor is being so unhelpful that his visits are detrimental to a patient. If a patient complains about a member of the clergy, or becomes anxious and upset whenever he visits, and the nurse cannot establish satisfactory communication with him, the nurse should discuss the matter with the hospital chaplain. He can investigate the situation and take appropriate action.

If a patient has no church affiliation or comes from out of town, the hospital chaplain provides another resource for spiritual help. Like the nurse, the chaplain's home turf is the hospital. Representing the church in a broad sense, the chaplain may be highly skilled in counseling and supporting ill persons and their families. A self-directed schedule enables the chaplain to spend large amounts of concentrated time with a few patients or brief moments with many, depending on his interests and style of ministry. Chaplains' departments and individual chaplains vary in their approach to patients and services offered. Nurses should get to know what their hospital provides as well as the chaplain and his staff.

Table 8. Comparison of Nurses and Clergy in Spiritual Care

Variables	Nurses	Clergy
Availability	**Daily eight-hour shift** Present at time of crisis or increased stress. Responsible for many patients, may have to interrupt conversation to tend others.	**Occasional visits** Seldom at the scene when crises occur. Able to concentrate full attention on person during visit.
Involvement	**Short-term and intensive** Unfamiliar with past history other than what is on patient's chart or what patient reveals. Knows only the family members who visit. May be less threatening, so patient can show doubts, fears, weakness. Relationship ends with discharge. Nature of task requires physical and emotional intimacy.	**Long-term and extensive** Has known patient prior to illness and during past crises. Knows family and family dynamics. Patient may feel embarrassed to show weakness, express doubts. Has continuing relationship. Usually relates to parishioner from "public zone."
Education and experience	**Nursing and nursing care** Focuses on health and illness. Theological understanding may be limited to personal beliefs. Understands the dynamics of illness and its effect on emotions; knows characteristics of specific illnesses.	**Theology and pastoral care** Focuses on spiritual growth and development. Understands patient's religious framework and can relate accordingly. Has limited understanding of the disease process; may be confused by illness or drug-related behavior.
Context and authority	**Hospital community** Hospital is "home turf"; experiences relative comfort with environment and illness; not usually overwhelmed by patient's condition; knows patient only in the context of his illness. Represents the hospital community; spiritual intervention is exercise of "priesthood of all believers."	**Church community** Hospital is foreign soil; may feel intimidated by atmosphere and equipment; disturbed by illness, especially if formerly healthy person is disfigured or disabled. Represents God and the church; spiritual intervention carries official status—can offer Communion.

Chapter 9
The Nurse's Personal Spiritual Resources

I can't.
I know that I must but
I can't.
It's part of the job
It has to be done
They say "go ahead" but
I can't.

I can't.
His light's on again but
I can't
Go in to that man
To suction him out
I'll surely be sick if I do
I can't.

Dear Lord
You love him I bet but
I can't.
Take my weak stomach
Hold me together
And give him your love through my care
I can't.

Linda J. Brobst, R.N.

F ive call lights glowed down the gloomy corridor as Sue Allison got off the elevator to take charge of the 3-11 shift. It was 2:45 P.M. but it seemed that work had already ceased for the day shift. The entire staff was lined up like a row of pigeons at the nurses' station, gazing past the call lights to focus on the minute hand of the clock as it slowly crept around to three o'clock. The ward secretary looked up to say, "Both the L.P.N. and the two aides called in sick this afternoon. The nursing office can't promise any replacements. Good luck!"

The patient in the room next to the nurses' station was rattling his side rails and moaning, "Help me." He expressed Sue's feelings exactly. She took a deep breath and hung up her coat.

"This place is lit up like a Christmas tree! Isn't anyone going to answer those lights?" Sue challenged the staff.

"Nope, I'm done for the day," replied Mary Beth, an R.N., as she removed her cap.

Sue felt exasperated and turned to the staff who remained, "Well, there's four of you and one of me. We can each answer one light."

As the day-shift personnel moved slowly back into action, Sue went into the room of the moaning patient. "What can I do for you, Mr. Whitaker?" Sue asked.

Mr. Whitaker's eyes darted frantically around the room, then rested on Sue. "I'm afraid. I'm all alone," he whispered. "Why has God deserted me like this?" "Deserted" seemed to describe Mr. Whitaker's condition well. He lay in a wad of wet linen. Urine trickled from his nephrostomy drain. His dressing lay on the floor by his bed. Sue applied a fresh dressing and quickly changed the linen.

"I'll be back right after report and rounds, Mr. Whitaker. We can talk then, okay?"

An abundance of extra personnel arrived during report. With a well-staffed unit, Sue felt she could spend some extra time with Mr. Whitaker. She kept her word to him and returned at 3:30.

Sue sat down beside Mr. Whitaker's bed. "You were saying you feel alone and afraid. What frightens you most?"

Mr. Whitaker closed his eyes and whispered, "Death."

Sue waited for him to continue.

After a brief silence he repeated, "Death . . . that's an awfully lonely feeling. And where is God in all of this?"

Sue was surprised. Mr. Whitaker wasn't dying. He had been admitted with a kidney stone last week. It had been removed surgically two days ago. He was recovering well; however, the severity of his pain, the experience of surgery and the sight of urine coming from his nephrostomy drain frightened Mr. Whitaker and confronted him with the possibility of death. He suddenly felt a desperate need to know God was with him and cared about him.

Sue responded to Mr. Whitaker's spiritual needs with sensitivity and skill over the next two days. By the time her days off arrived she felt exhausted and empty. Besides the physical fatigue from working ten days without a break, she also felt guilty that she had not been more sensitive to Mr. Whitaker's spiritual needs earlier in his hospitalization. The thought struck her that she had considered Mr. Whitaker to be only a "routine kidney stone" who needed minimal attention. The four patients on respirators, the sixteen with I.V.'s, and the two patients in isolation had consumed most of Sue's time and energy. Sue was angry with herself for violating her own convictions about caring for the whole person. She knew spiritual needs were important, but with Mr. Whitaker she had failed to recognize them, much less meet them, until he became desperate.

Sue was experiencing "burn out," a common problem of people in the helping professions.[1] Nurses can only continue to meet the needs of other people if their own needs are being met. Unless we are constantly refueled, spiritual care can be so personally draining that we either collapse in exhaustion or withdraw from the people who need us.

How can we avoid burn out? To begin with, we need to recognize that compulsive need-meeting is not a virtue. It is actually an overestimation of our self-importance. God can use other people just as easily as he can use us in meeting a person's spiritual needs. Each of us also has the responsibility to maintain optimum physical, psychosocial and spiritual health in our own lives as well as in our patients'. Nurses, like patients, are integrated beings. We need proper rest, exercise and diet to function at our best. Let us review our working definition of man and see its application to us as nurses:

Man is a physically, psychosocially and spiritually integrated being. . . .

Sue Allison had worked eight hectic days in a row when we met her at the beginning of this chapter. Fatigue limited her ability to perceive the spiritual and emotional needs of her patients even though ordinarily she was quite sensitive. She was also confronted with interpersonal tensions among the nursing personnel which drained her energy. As human beings we need a sense of belonging and togetherness, of support and encouragement from our peers. We need to experience the love and concern of others for us before we can pass this on to patients.

We also need spiritual strength. Sue had been so tired from work that she had neglected her times of personal prayer and Bible study. She had also been unable to attend church services on Sunday because she had worked 7-3. Nurses, as well as patients, have spiritual needs. Those needs must be met before we can function at an optimum level.

That we are integrated beings means that unmet need in one area of our lives affects our total being. One of the first steps we can take to avoid burn out is to plan a balanced schedule so that we have time for rest, relaxation, worship, a variety of social activities and a personal support system as well as work. Setting measurable goals, in writing, is helpful for maintaining balance and providing a troubleshooter's guide when things seem to be going wrong. Table 9 gives some major areas we should consider in setting our goals.

Man is . . . created to live in harmony with God. . . .

The whole point of this book is that we are created to live in harmony with God, and *because of that fact* nurses must provide spiritual care for patients. We cannot give away what we do not possess. We ourselves must be in harmony with God before we can begin to assist patients spiritually. What does it mean to live in harmony with God? A nurse who has begun to find out shares some of her insights with us:

Graduation day catapulted me from the role of learner to performer.

Table 9. Areas to Consider in Setting Personal Goals

Physical	Weight
	Grooming
	Sleep
	Exercise
	Diet
	Routine medical and dental examinations
Psychosocial	Supportive relationships
	Socialization
	Hobbies
	Cultural enrichment
	Community involvement
	Professional growth
	Intellectual stimulation
	Relaxation
Spiritual	Personal prayer and Bible study
	Prayer partner
	Small group fellowship
	Church affiliation

As a visiting nurse I found myself responsible for an area which included part of Greenwich Village, Little Italy, Chinatown and the Wall Street area. This position was planned to prepare me for a Peace Corps assignment which I refused when I learned it was to be in Afghanistan. The prospect of two years of rural living made me realize the limits of my idealism. My pride would not allow me to return to the Visiting Nurse Service where I had been given a farewell party. I sought a job in a local hospital and became head nurse on a surgical unit. I coped with my responsibility by spending twelve hours a day on my work. The long hours, my tension headaches, and a growing bitterness made me wonder if the rewards of responsibility justified the cost. I submitted my resignation and converted my savings account into travelers checks and an around-the-world airline ticket. My trip consisted of 32 stops to be completed in 80 days. I limited the time to 80 days because I had met a man whom I thought I would marry. Marriage itself did not excite me; I thought that after I had "seen the world" I would be more willing to "settle down."

My travels satisfied my need for adventure at the expense of an ever-increasing loneliness. I was an outsider wherever I went. Relationships formed with men and women were transient. Despair set in. I disregarded my earlier plans and endeavored only to feel good. In a short time I became physically ill and a place to rest became a priority. Someone told me about a ski resort in the Swiss Alps where I could stay without charge for 10 days. The prospect was appealing enough to make me travel across Switzerland and up a mountain in search of the place. To my delight the people I found there spoke English, but to my dismay it was not a ski resort, but a religious commune. I was surprised to find the people there to be rather intelligent and more knowledgeable than myself about modern philosophers. Their apparent interest in my well-being I found unnerving. I was intrigued enough to stay, although I winced at the prospect of sharing a bedroom with 11 girls and a bathroom with 25.

I enjoyed the view and the food and remained on the periphery of things until I was cornered by an English hippy who asked me pointed questions about my belief or lack of belief in God. We talked until 3:15 in the morning and for the first time I thought it might be logical to believe in a personal God. I read a book by Francis Schaeffer, The God Who Is There, and Clark Pinnock's book, Set Forth Your Case, and thought about the emptiness of my own life. I realized that no matter what I did, I could not feel satisfied. I realized one night by myself on a mountainside that the time had come to make a choice . . . and I committed my life to Christ.

I felt a tremendous uplift and a new joy. I made the decision to stay at L'Abri [the name of the commune] for three months. Doubt set in and I decided that it was the place and the people who were responsible for my new sense of peace. I set out alone again, traveling through Germany and Italy questioning people on planes and buses, in discotheques, pensiones and hotels as to what was their reason for living. Simultaneously I decided to relate to God as if He were a person and expected tangible signs of His presence. Within a month I decided that Jesus was in fact God and I flew home to New York.

I was a bundle of excitement, feeling that I had found the meaning of life. The God of creation must have smiled. . . . I told everyone about Jesus and worked harder than ever to be a good nurse—for life had meaning. I exhausted myself and wound up in the hospital with viral *pneumonia. There, in a new way, I found that I could let go and let God. I have a new peace and a new joy, perhaps because I am learning from experience that I can trust Jesus. Because I can trust Him, I am more obedient to Him. For a time I thought that my quest was over because I had found "the Answer." Instead, I have found Jesus who is gently guiding me through life.* [2]

The first step toward living in harmony with God is recognizing Jesus Christ as the Lord of life and redeemer from sin. This recognition may take place suddenly or develop over a lifetime, but it is an absolute prerequisite to life in harmony with God. Once a commitment to Christ is established, a relationship with him continues to develop as we spend time in Bible study, prayer and fellowship with other Christians.

The Bible has been described as "God's love letter to man." Through studying the Bible we learn of God's personal concern for us and for the world. We get to know more about God's character. The more we know about God, the more we will be able to trust him. Bible study is a personal resource for nurses because from Scripture we can view the world and our problems from God's perspective.

The Bible is a source of strength and refreshment. We need to spend time each day studying it to remain spiritually strong and vibrant. Numerous guides for personal Bible study have been developed. Appendix C offers some suggestions. We should try to set aside a period of time each day for personal Bible study and prayer, making it a top priority in our schedule.

Prayer is our response to God—a response of worship, praise, thanksgiving, confession, intercession and petition. It is a verbal recognition of our humanity and our need for God. It is saying, "I can't, but God can through me." It is a vital link with our source of strength.

Prayer does not have to be reserved for quiet, formal occasions. It is an on-the-spot resource as well. Many nurses have found that praying silently for a patient as they walk down the hall to answer his light generally enables them to hear more accurately what the patient is trying to say when they get to his room. Prayer helps us respond more appropriately to patients' needs, and prayer keeps things in perspective. It is easy for a sensitive nurse to become overinvolved with a patient and take on too much personal responsibility for the patient's recovery. Stopping to pray serves to remind us that we are not God and that God himself is able to care for that patient far beyond our limited time and ability.

Affiliation with a local church and regular participation in its worship and other activities are also important resources for maintaining harmony with God. Becoming involved in the worship, educational programs and social activities of a congregation provides support, encouragement and stimulation in our growth as Christians. We should find some way we can contribute to the life of our church—by doing such things as teaching, visiting, singing or joining a study group. We should get to know our minister and share with him our joys and struggles in nursing. We will probably be a great encouragement to him as he becomes a support for us.

Another helpful resource is a "prayer partner." We should find someone with whom we can share mutual concerns regularly, then pray about them together. It may be someone at work, or someone from our church or fellowship group.

Our relationship with God is our basic personal resource in the spiritual care of patients. If our spiritual intervention is based on any other foundation than a commitment to Jesus Christ as Lord and Savior, we can only set up ourselves, or some nebulous force, as God. We end up making feelings our ultimate authority. To do so provides a shaky source of security at a time when both the patient and the nurse need stability. We find our stability through a life lived in harmony with God.

Man is . . . created to live in harmony with . . . himself. . . .

Nurses are not immune to suffering. Past experiences, both the joyous and the tragic ones, are personal resources for us. Living in harmony with ourselves requires coming to grips with both the positive and negative experiences in our lives. Personal suffering may be one of the most meaningful ways we can learn to understand and empathize with our patients.

We grow from the suffering we experience. The diary of a nurse with multiple sclerosis illustrates this painful growth process at work:

Sept. 12: *I long to talk with people around me. I want to cry with them near me. Yet, I can't reach out to them. Oh, how I long for them to come to me. How I wish they would let me know, somehow, that they understand. I wrestle alone.*

Sept. 13: *I was very lonely today. Last night I cried myself to sleep. Other nights I could not sleep at all. I knew God was near, but I didn't feel his nearness.*

Sept. 14: *Flashing through my mind today came many patients I have cared for. They also must have been waiting and struggling alone. They, too, must have wanted someone to reach out to them—someone to express caring without having to be asked first. They probably needed to talk about "it"—even as I need to talk. My insides are churning. I wonder how often I have made patients handle their fears and loneliness by themselves, because I was afraid of the pain of struggling with them. How often have I been completely oblivious to what their needs might be? How many times have I heard a patient giving me a double message about how he was feeling, but ignored it? I probably thought it would be too personal, or too nosy, to explore it. That was a cop-out. More than likely, I was afraid to get too involved. How I long to retrace some steps—to go back and tell them that now I understand.*

Sept. 15: *To live with sorrow seething within is like living in the valley of a mountain that constantly threatens to erupt. It is fearing that the hot lava will not only destroy a portion of the mountain itself, but also destroy any person who gets in its path. I sit, afraid to involve anyone too deeply in my fight. I sit in the valley, afraid of the volcano erupting.*

Sept. 16: *I have one friend who is not afraid of the hot lava. Dorrit waits with me, prays with me, and allows the eruption to happen—even encourages it to happen. Strangely, as the fiery mixture pours out it has a cauterizing effect on portions of a gaping, hurting wound. Slowly, I have begun to realize that healing has begun. Dorrit makes no demands —only that I tell her what hurts and why. Then she gathers me in her arms and lets me weep. It seems that weeping has become an attitude of life for me, and she understands my sorrow. Although she allows me my mood-swings and preoccupation with myself, she gently nudges me into "the now." She does not push me there to struggle alone; rather, she extends her hand, and her heart, and walks with me. She takes me with her in prayer, too, when I feel I can't stand before the throne of God alone. It was good to see Dorrit today.*

Jan. 25: *My sorrow has turned into seething anger. It is God that I am angry with—even though I take it out on myself and other people.*

For weeks I have been saying "this should never happen to me," but today I'm suddenly struck by the fact that it has happened to me. The battle raged so fierce inside me today that I screamed at God and told him that I have had enough. Then I sobbed for hours and told God everything—my anger, my fears, my conflicts. God had not forsaken me, I had forsaken him. I feel rotten.

Jan. 26: I am learning something new about how God accepts me where I am. He loves me in spite of how I feel or what I think.

Feb. 1: Today I looked into the mirror and didn't recognize myself. The fluid has collected in the tissues of my body, my face is puffy, my clothes don't fit, it's hard to breathe. I feel like the real me has already died, only fragments remain, and those fragments don't look familiar. I went to work but it all seemed fruitless, I just couldn't produce. I want to find a secluded place and sit there. I couldn't stand being with groups of people today. I am repulsed by myself and expect others to feel the same way. It is frightening to see my whole personality changing. I hate being related to me. I'm so tired!

Five years later: Writing what I did kept me sane. Writing it down, and seeing it, and knowing I was still alive and communicating with someone, even though it was myself, helped me to see who I was and what I needed. It has been valuable beyond all measure.[3]

Most of us have not suffered as extensively or intensively as the person who wrote this diary, but each of us has experienced some form of loss, separation, failure or crisis. It is a human tendency to repress painful experiences, leaving a gnawing sense of anger, pain or guilt. Prayerfully examining those experiences can give a personal sense of peace as well as provide insights into the needs of patients. A quick evaluation of what you have learned about yourself, God and other people through past experiences can be constructive. Who was helpful when you were in a crisis? How did they help? How did you feel? What did you do with your feelings? How did the crisis affect your relationship with God?

If you find that thinking about past experiences stirs up emotions which were not adequately resolved at the time of the crisis, you may need help in working through those feelings now. A trusted friend or minister may be a helpful person to support you by listening and praying with you. Professional counseling may be necessary for deep-seated struggles. Our effectiveness in helping others is, to a large extent, dependent on how well we have coped with our own difficulties.

Man is . . . created to live in harmony . . . with . . . others.

New town, new job, new friends—what had seemed so exciting to Steve in June now added up to loneliness and frustration. The big city which had lured him by its call to adventure, experience and excitement now added up to tripled car insurance rates, an alcoholic head nurse who delighted in announcing her staff's mistakes to patients and co-workers, and a church group where no one could remember his name. "I want to give nursing a fair try, but after my first six months, I sure don't like it!" Steve thought to himself. He longed for someone to talk to.

Mary first dared to pray with a patient last month. Her patient's burns had become overwhelming for both of them. As she changed his dressing, he cried out in pain and Mary joined him in tears. In despair she said, "The only thing I know to help is prayer." She prayed aloud for him and watched him relax for the first time in days. While that experience encouraged Mary to become involved with her patients spiritually, she also found it was draining. Her level of commitment to this patient was higher than she could afford to give to everyone. How could she set priorities for spiritual intervention? She sensed a need for advice and prayer support from other Christians.

Jim arrived home from the state nurses' convention enthused and troubled at the same time. He had been elected Second Vice-president of the State Nurses Association but found he could not endorse some of the issues the association was supporting. He felt alone in a secular world, needing prayer and active involvement with Christian nurses who could understand his plight.

Alma is teaching medical-surgical nursing in a university program. This week she helped nursing students begin a Bible study. She is tired of educational politics and hassles and wants to use her time for the Lord, so she may leave nursing entirely to be an evangelist with a home mission board.

The list could go on and on—nurses who are alienated within the profession.[4] Nurses who are involved in spiritual care and implementing Christian principles need a support system. We need other people who understand our situation and are able to support and encourage us. We need to be able to share with one another. Some nurses will be able to find that kind of support within their local churches, but others have found a nurses' fellowship group especially meaningful and helpful. Suggestions are provided in the appendix if you would like help in finding, or forming, a nurses' fellowship group.

We were created to live in harmony with other people. We cannot operate for very long in isolation from other people, or in opposition to other people, before we run out of steam. The love and support of others is an energizing force. Harmony with others involves giving and receiving forgiveness, talking over disagreements and constructively handling anger and frustration. Living in harmony with others enables us to channel our energy into the fulfillment of the meaning and purpose of our lives. Harmonious relationships with other people are a basic spiritual resource for nurses.

Nurses are physically, psychosocially and spiritually integrated beings, created to live in harmony with God, themselves and others.

Our personal spiritual resources are basically the same resources we offer to our patients. We cannot deal with our spiritual needs in isolation from our physical and psychosocial needs. We must see ourselves as whole persons, just as we view our patients.

Our effectiveness as helping people is dependent on the harmony we experience with God, ourselves and other people. We need a confident sense of meaning and purpose in our own lives in order to assist our patients in finding meaning and purpose in their illness and in their lives. We need to experience the love of God and other people in order to love our patients. We need to know personal forgiveness from God and others in order to communicate forgiveness to our patients. Spiritual needs—both our own and our patients'—are met by God, who communicates his meaning and purpose, his love, and his forgiveness to us through prayer, Scripture and other people.

Appendix A
Spiritual Needs Research

Spiritual Needs Survey
Compiled by Jean Stallwood Hess, R.N., M.S.N.
Spring 1969

A pilot project was conducted by Nurses Christian Fellowship to determine patients' awareness of their spiritual needs. Twelve nurses affiliated with Nurses Christian Fellowship interviewed one hundred nine papatients in hospitals and extended care facilities in various parts of the United States. Patients chosen for the study met these criteria: eighteen years old or older; not in a critical phase of illness; hospitalized three days or longer. Religion or denominational affiliation was not considered as a criterion, but hospital records indicated this sampling:

Sampling	Number of Patients
Nonsectarian health facility	71
Sectarian health facility	38
Protestant	73
Roman Catholic	24
Jewish	6
No affiliation	6
Women	60
Men	49
Age range	18-90 years
Medical diagnosis	67
Surgical diagnosis	42

These questions were asked:

1. Were you aware of having a spiritual need at any time during your hospitalization?
2. Are you able to describe it and can you tell me about it?
3. With whom did you discuss this need?
4. How did you feel about the assistance you received?
5. Has your need been met to any degree or is it still present?

In response to the first question, the need for prayer was most frequently expressed—to pray personally, to be prayed for or to pray with another person. Comments included "I can't pray; my prayers aren't heard"; "I couldn't have gotten along without prayer"; "I prayed constantly because I was sure I was dying."

Loneliness was also mentioned as was the need for an awareness of God's presence. One patient commented, "I feel so lonesome and discouraged about my health that I'm about to give up." Another stated a need for the assurance of God's presence and help.

Approximately 18% of the participants described a fear of surgery and death, and, for the men in particular, a need to find meaning and purpose in life, death and suffering. Feelings of guilt, loss of faith and doubt were also mentioned in addition to the need to express faith by visible and tangible means such as Bible reading, Holy Communion, church attendance and the lighting of candles.

Patients also expressed a desire for assistance from a hospital chaplain, minister, priest or rabbi. These spiritual counselors were the most frequently mentioned persons in response to the third question, "With whom did you discuss this need?" Nurses ranked second, followed by family members, friends, a psychiatrist, other hospital personnel or roommate, and God. Of those interviewed, 87 referred to help from other people, 4 mentioned the Bible and/or prayer, and 11 said they received no help at all. Patients who did not wish to discuss their spiritual need, or were unable to, made these comments: "I don't want help"; "I don't know where to turn"; "I could never talk to a clergyman"; "I can take care of my own need."

In response to question 4, "How did you feel about the assistance you received?" answers ranged from "It was exactly what I needed" to "It was of no help." However, the majority of replies were positive.

The majority of patients interviewed also said that though their spiritual need had been met to some degree it was still present.

A sixth question, not a part of the original interview but asked when appropriate, was, "How do you think nurses might help patients meet spiritual needs?" The responses below were categorized and are typical of the majority view:

Too Busy

"I really feel nurses are too busy to give much time to this, unfortunately."

"They are too busy. . . . If . . . they really cared, that might help as much as a minister."

"I wouldn't bother the nurse with such things. They're too busy; they don't have time to stop and talk or listen. I wish they did though."

Unsure

"I think they could, but I don't know how."

Not Their Duty

"I don't feel they should unless asked by a patient."

"Out of their line of work. Chaplain should take care of spiritual needs."

How Nurses Can Help

"Listen."

"Recognize a need and contact the chaplain."

" . . . enter into the conversation with us."

"Pray with patients and take time to talk."

"Being alert and watching for their particular need; then being sympathetic enough to know what to say. In my case, I found talking and making me understand was enough."

" . . . don't hesitate to discuss religious matters."

"By tactfully asking questions and then seeking outside help if needed."

One conclusion drawn from this study was that many patients would appreciate help in meeting their spiritual needs from a nurse who was available to listen and then personally intervene or refer to the appropriate spiritual counselor. A nurse should also be sensitive to the patient who believes that spiritual care is not the nurse's role and the patient who desires no help at all.

Spiritual Needs of Patients Study
Claire Martin, R.N.; Cherill Burrows, R.N.; Jane Pomilio, R.N.
State University of New York at Utica-Rome
School of Nursing, Upper Division
May 1976

Methodology

Research Design. The investigators of this empirical descriptive study of spiritual needs of patients elected the survey method as the most appropriate way to collect data from hospitalized persons. A questionnaire was designed because of its economy and ease of distribution. Primarily nominal data were sought, although some ordinal ranking was requested; and the questionnaire best suited this purpose. The possible low return rate of questionnaires was considered. The investigators personally handed the questionnaires to the subjects with an explanation of the purpose of the study in an effort to stimulate a higher return. Questionnaires were collected the same day, one day later or two days later with a request to interview the patient at that time. It was felt that the interview would enhance the findings on the questionnaires and allow the investigators to gather personal information from the subjects. The investigators were aware of the possibility of the Hawthorne effect and attempted to control this by carefully monitoring their reactions and responses to the patient.

Sample. The participants in the study were selected from the adult population of two area general hospitals. This convenience sample numbered 90 participants—49 males and 41 females. Their selection met the criteria of availability, voluntary participation, rationality and noncritical status.

Instruments and procedure. Data were collected from patients using two instruments: a questionnaire and an interview schedule. Participants were asked to complete the questionnaire; then an investigator returned to the bedside to conduct the interview. The questionnaire was preceded by an explanatory paragraph stating the purpose of the study and that participation in the survey was voluntary and anonymous. There were three sections to the questionnaire. Section I elicited demographic data such as age, sex, marital status and church affiliation of the participant. Section II contained 10 statements about the spiritual dimension of care.

The respondent was asked to indicate degree of agreement or disagreement with the statement on a 5-point Likert scale. Eight statements specifically related spiritual care to nursing behavior and patients' perceptions of nurses' attitudes and qualifications to administer spiritual care. These statements were chosen because they were representative of the patient responses reported in the 1969 Nurses Christian Fellowship study on spiritual needs of patients. Section III of the questionnaire consisted of two items. Item 1 contained a list of 7 types of spiritual needs reported most often in the Nurses Christian Fellowship and Weiler studies. The participant was asked to rank these according to importance to him. Item 2 was a list of 8 possible nursing interventions. Patients were asked to indicate which they believed to be appropriate ways a nurse could give spiritual care:

Sample Questionnaire

This is a questionnaire designed to determine the spiritual needs that hospitalized persons experience. As we have cared for people who are ill, we have become aware that some of their needs do not seem to be met. So, in conjunction with a nursing course at Upper Division College, we are asking patients to answer these questions. Participation in this survey is completely voluntary. We ask that you state honestly how you feel about any spiritual need you have felt, any spiritual care you have received, and what role the nurses may have had in your spiritual care. No names will be taken so your answers will remain anonymous. Your answers and comments will be appreciated and given careful attention. The information that you supply will be used to help improve the quality and expand the scope of nursing care. If you do not wish to participate, would you mind sharing your reason with us? If you are willing to participate, please continue with the survey. Thank you for your assistance.
Cherill Burrows, R.N., Claire Martin, R.N., Jane Pomilio, R.N.
Upper Division College Nursing Dept.

Spiritual Needs of Patients Study
Questionnaire

Section 1
Instructions: Please fill in the blanks with the appropriate information.
Age_____ Sex_____ Marital Status_____ Occupation_____
Church Affiliation_____
How many times have you been hospitalized in the past 5 years?_____
Is anyone helping you to fill out this questionnaire?_____
If yes, please specify_____

Section 2

Instructions: Please circle the x under the column that best describes how you feel about the statement on the corresponding line.

	strongly agree	agree	undecided	disagree	strongly disagree
1. A person who is ill thinks more about his relationship to God.	x	x	x	x	x
2. Nurses are not qualified to help patients meet their spiritual needs.	x	x	x	x	x
3. A nurse should ask every patient if he/she wishes to see a clergyman.	x	x	x	x	x
4. Nurses give spiritual care by being concerned, cheerful, and kind.	x	x	x	x	x
5. I would appreciate a visit from a clergyman but would not request it unless someone suggested it.	x	x	x	x	x
6. A patient's beliefs about God are too personal to discuss with the nurse.	x	x	x	x	x
7. Nurses are too busy to help patients with their spiritual needs.	x	x	x	x	x
8. I would enjoy having a nurse read me the Scriptures, or pray with me.	x	x	x	x	x
9. Nurses who talk about God with patients are trying to convert them.	x	x	x	x	x
10. A nurse who sits down and listens is helping me spiritually.	x	x	x	x·	x

Section 3

1. Instructions: The following types of spiritual needs have been expressed by hospitalized persons. Using the numbers 1 to 7, please rank them in order of importance to you, 1 being most important and descending in order to 7 being least important to you.

———— Relief from fear of death   ———— Purpose and meaning in life
———— Visit from a clergyman   ———— Expression of caring and support
———— Prayer   from another person
———— Knowledge of God's presence   ———— Sacraments, communion

2. Instructions: Please place a check mark in front of the following statements that you feel are appropriate ways a nurse may give spiritual care to patients.

———— Refer patient to a clergyman
———— Pray with a patient
———— Talk with a patient about God and religious beliefs
———— Read Scriptures to a patient
———— Show kindness, concern, and cheerfulness when giving care
———— Listen to a patient talk about God and his religious beliefs
———— Encourage the patient to talk about anything that is bothering him
———— Obtain Scriptures or other religious material for the patient
———— Other

The interview schedule consisted of these questions:

1. Were you aware of having a spiritual need at any time during your hospitalization? Are you able to describe this need and can you tell me about it?

2. With whom did you discuss this need?

3. How did you feel about the assistance you received?

4. Has your need been met to any degree or is it still present?

5. How often do you usually attend church?

6. How do you think nurses might help patients meet spiritual needs?

Question 5 on the frequency of church attendance was asked to determine if it bore any relationship to the number or type of spiritual needs experienced by hospitalized persons. The interview schedule was the same one used in the Nurses Christian Fellowship study with 109 patients. The questionnaire was designed specifically for this study and was not pretested.

Statistical methodology. Findings of this study will be reported as raw data, as percentages of defined categories, as descriptive statistics such as modes and means, and in the nonparametric z value for an obtained sum of ranks for a Mann-Whitney U test. Because this data obtained in this study are nominal and ordinal, a nonparametric statistic is appropriate. In Section II, the Likert opinion responses to 8 of the questions were assigned a positional value reflecting degree of positive and negative feelings toward the need for spiritual care and delivery of that care by a nurse. The range of possible scores is 8-40. Scores of 32-40 indicate a strong positive opinion regarding need for spiritual care and the nurse's role in providing that care. Scores of 16 or below reflect a strong negative stance by the subject. Those scores ranging between 16 and 32 indicate less definite and consistent opinions with scores over 24 tending to be more positive and those under 24 more negative. The individual scores for each group tested are rank ordered, assigned ranks, and the sum of the ranks is the statistic used to calculate the z score for the Mann-Whitney U statistic. Since all the samples in this study are large, it will not be necessary to calculate the U; but the z score itself can determine the significance of differences between groups. The 95% confidence level (.05 significance level) determines the acceptable critical value for our purpose.

Findings

All 90 subjects completed the questionnaire; 65 subjects agreed to be interviewed as well. There were 49 male subjects (54%) and 41 females (46%). Of the participants 64% were married, 13% were single, 14% were widowed, 7% were separated or divorced, 2% did not respond. The age range of the subjects was 16 to 87 years. The mean age was 53.8 years. There was a modal frequency of 23 in the 50-59 year range. Forty-eight per cent of the subjects were Catholic, 42% Protestant, 8% claimed no church affiliation and 2% did not respond to that question. Protestant denominations represented among the subjects were Methodist, Presbyterian, Episcopal, Baptist, Holiness and Lutheran. Of the survey participants, 27% were hospitalized one time during the prior 5 years; 23% were hospitalized 2 times in the past 5 years; 49% were hospitalized 3 or more times, and 1% did not respond. Data regarding occupations of the subjects were inconsistently reported so that analysis of that variable was not meaningful as being representative.

Interview. Of the 65 patients interviewed, 31 were women and 34 were men. In responding to question 1, "Were you aware of having a spiritual need at any time during your hospitalization? Are you able to describe this need and can you tell me about it?" 48% (31) said they did experience a spiritual need while hospitalized and 52% (34) stated they did not. Sixty-eight per cent of those persons verbalizing a spiritual need were women (21 of the 31). The remaining 32% (10) were men. Half the male respondents did not specify the nature of their spiritual need or stated it was too personal to share. Those needs that men did express were for support, hope, help, conversation, a relationship to God and freedom from discouragement. Only 2 female respondents would not reveal the kind of spiritual need they experienced. The following list points out the variety of spiritual needs that were shared by the women: relief from nervousness, worry, fear, loneliness; concern for husband and children; fear of tests and diagnosis; knowledge of God's presence and relatedness; need for calmness, comfort, salvation, help; desire to see a clergyman; communion; reason for suffering.

Table 1. *Male/Female Distribution of Subjects (Question 1)*

	Total	Total Per cent	Frequency Male	Per cent Male	Frequency Female	Per cent Female
Subjects	65	100%	34	52%	31	48%
Have spiritual need	31	48%	10	32%	21	68%
No spiritual need	34	52%	24	71%	10	29%
Named spiritual need	24	77%	5	21%	19	79%
Spiritual need not named	7	23%	5	71%	2	28%

Question 2. "With whom did you discuss this need?" Twenty (65%) of the 31 people who experienced a spiritual need talked with one or more people about it. Of the 20, 13 were women and 7 were men. The clergyman was most frequently named as the confidante people used.

Others named were family members, the nurse, friends, the doctor and God. Patients who denied having a spiritual need were asked who they would discuss this need with were it present. They named the same persons listed in Table 2.

Table 2. Persons with Whom Patients Discussed This Need (Question 2)		Table 3. Feelings of Patients after Receiving Assistance (Question 3)	
Person Consulted	Number of Patients	Feeling	Number of Patients
Clergyman	16	More positive	2
Family	5	Good, better	13
Nurse	4	Ambivalent	1
Friend	3	Comforted	1
Doctor	2	Helped	3
God only	3	Not helped	3
Total	33*		

Total N = 20
*Some patients discussed need with more than one person.

Question 3. "How did you feel about the assistance you received?" The most frequent response to this question was "good" or "better." One respondent said it helped to talk with someone but the problem was not solved. Table 3 shows the range of responses.

Question 4. "Has your need been met to any degree or is it still present?" Of the respondents, 48% stated that their needs were completely met, 16% said they were partly met, and 29% indicated they were not met. Table 4 presents this data.

Question 5. "How often do you usually attend church?" Responses to this question were classified according to frequency of church attendance. The three categories used were (1) regularly, (2) occasionally and (3) rarely or never. Regular attendance was defined as attending church one or more times per week. Occasional attendance applied to subjects attending church less than once a week but at least once every six weeks. The rarely/never category included all those attending less often than once every six weeks. The sample included approximately the same number of subjects in each group with the similar distribution by sex.

Table 4. Degree to Which Needs Were Met (Question 4)			Table 5. Church Attendance (Question 5)			
	Number	Per cent		Regular	Occasional	R/N*
Completely	15	48.4%	Female	11	10	10
Partly	5	16.1%	Male	9	14	11
Not at all	9	29.0%				
No response	2	6.5%				
Total	31	100%	Total	20	24	21
			*R/N: rarely/never			

Question 6. "How do you think nurses might help patients meet spiritual needs?" This question received responses from 41 people. Some respondents made several suggestions. The response that occurred most often was one that indicated the respondent would like the nurse to listen to whatever the patient needed to talk about. The second most frequent response was that the nurse could call the patient's clergy-

Table 6. Nursing Interventions Deemed Appropriate by Patients (Question 6)

Description of Nurse's Activity	**Response Frequency**
Listen to patient, allow patient to talk	24
Call clergyman	13
Be pleasant, kind, polite	10
Be understanding	7
Read Scripture to patient	6
Be caring, comforting, encouraging	5
"Be there"	4
Give good care	3
Ask patient's wishes and comply	2
Talk about God to patient	2
Build patient's ego	1
Remain hopeful	1
Pray with patient	1
Be alert to patient's needs	1
Explain procedures	1
Other Comments	
Don't have enough time	8
Nurses can't help in this area	6
It's not their job	3
Don't know	2

man if the patient requested it. Some subjects said that nurses do not have time to help with spiritual needs or that it is not their job. The two most negative responses were that most nurses will not respond to a patient's requests and that "sometimes you can't even get them to come to your room." Table 6 displays the data collected on this question.

Questionnaire. Ninety subjects completed parts or all of the three-section questionnaire. Section I dealt with demographic data and those data have already been reported.

Data from Section II will be handled in two ways. First, an overview of patients' responses will be presented by reporting the calculated percentages of subjects agreeing or disagreeing with the statements. Second, the results of the Mann-Whitney U statistic in the form of z scores will be used to test the null hypothesis that the set of measurements of one group is equal to another group. Groups tested were according to age, sex, religious affiliation, frequency of church attendance and frequency of hospitalization.

Table 7. Overview of Responses by Percentage of Total Responding

Statement	Agreed	Undecided	Disagreed
1	84%	8%	8%
2	35%	25%	40%
3	73%	9%	18%
4	97%	0%	3%
5	33%	11%	56%
6	41%	9%	50%
7	58%	16%	26%
8	13%	29%	58%
9	13%	9%	78%
10	77%	13%	10%

See Section II of questionnaire for content of statements.

Statement 1 read, "A person who is ill thinks more about his relationship with God." Of the subjects, 84% agreed with this statement.

Statement 2 read, "Nurses are not qualified to help patients meet their spiritual needs." The respondents were fairly evenly split on this question with 35% in agreement, 40% in disagreement and 25% undecided.

Statement 3 read, "A nurse should ask every patient if he/she wishes to see a clergyman." Those in agreement totaled 73% with 18% disagreeing.

Statement 4 read, "Nurses give spiritual care by being concerned, cheerful, and kind." A staggering 97% agreed with that statement.

Statement 5 was found to be ambiguous: "I would appreciate a visit from a clergyman but would not request it unless someone suggested it." Fifty-six per cent of the subjects disagreed and 33% agreed, but there is no way to determine whether the response applies to the first clause or the second.

Statement 6 read, "A patient's beliefs about God are too personal to discuss with the nurse." Once again there was a split, with 41% agreeing and 50% disagreeing.

Statement 7 read, "Nurses are too busy to help patients with their spiritual needs." While 58% of the participants agreed with that statement, 26% disagreed.

Statement 8 read, "I would enjoy having a nurse read me the Scriptures, or pray with me." The majority of the subjects (58%) disagreed while 29% were undecided.

Statement 9 read, "Nurses who talk about God with patients are trying to convert them." While 78% of the respondents disagreed with that item, those undecided totaled 9%.

Statement 10 read, "A nurse who sits down and listens is helping me spiritually." Here 77% agreed, 10% disagreed and 13% were undecided.

Responses to statements 2, 3, 4, 6, 7, 8, 9 and 10 were used as indicators of the patient's interest in hospital spiritual care and his perception of the nurse's role in providing that care. Regular churchgoers as a group were compared with occasional attenders and with those who rarely or never went to church. The occasional group was also tested with the rarely/never group. The z value for the regular/occasional ratio was .013; for the regular/rarely-never ratio, 1.12; and for the occasional/rarely-never ratio, 1.49. None of these values were significant and the

Table 8. Results of z Value for an Obtained Sum of Ranks for a Mann-Whitney U Test

Groups Compared	z	Groups Compared	z
Catholic/Protestant	.053	Age 39-/65+	2.73
Male/Female	3.16	39-/40→	1.46
Frequency of Hosp. once/more		40→/65+	.077
than 5 times in 5 years	2.71		
Frequency of Church Attendance		**Level of Significance**	
Reg/Occas	.013	for .05, z = 1.96	
Reg/Rare-Never	1.12	for .01, z = 2.58	
Occas/Rare-Never	1.49		

null hypothesis of equality between groups could not be rejected. Responses of the Catholic subjects were analyzed with those of the Protestants and the z=.053. Again the null hypothesis could not be rejected. Male/female categorical groups were tested and the responses were found to differ significantly at the .01 level. The z score was 3.16. Those patients hospitalized only one time in the prior five years were tested with those patients who had been hospitalized five times or more in the same time frame. The z score was 2.71, indicating a significant difference between groups at the .01 significance level. The sample was analyzed according to three age groups: those subjects 39 years of age and younger (39-), those participants in the 40-64 year range (40→), and those who were 65 years old or older (65+). The 39- group differed significantly from the 65+ group (z=2.73), but not from the 40→ group (z=1.46). The 40→ group did not vary significantly from the 65+ group (z=.077).

Table 9. Ranking of Spiritual Needs by Church Affiliation

Catholic	Protestant	Spiritual Need
1	6	Relief from fear of death
2	5	Visit from a clergyman
4	3	Prayer
5	1	Knowledge of God's presence
6	4	Purpose and meaning in life
7	2	Expression of caring and support from another person
3	7	Sacraments, communion

Ranking was done in accordance with order of importance to the patient.
N = 56

Table 10. Patients' Perceptions of Appropriate Nursing Interventions as Recorded by Subjects According to Church Affiliation

Intervention	Cath	Prot	None	Total	Per cent of N
1. Refer patient to clergyman	26	20	4	50	57%
2. Pray with patient	7	14	1	22	25%
3. Talk with patient about God	10	12	2	24	27%
4. Read Scriptures to patient	8	12	2	22	25%
5. Show kindness, concern, cheer	36	35	9	80	91%
6. Listen to patient talk re God	16	15	4	35	40%
7. Encourage patient to talk	29	32	7	68	77%
8. Obtain Scriptures for patient	8	12	1	21	24%

Total N = 88

Table 11. Patients' Perceptions of Appropriate Nursing Interventions as Recorded by Subjects According to Frequency of Church Attendance

Intervention Number	Total N	Per cent of N	Regular		Occasional		Rare/Never	
			f	%	f	%	f	%
1	42	47.7	15	17.0%	18	20.5%	9	10.2%
2	18	20.5	3	3.4%	10	11.4%	5	5.7%
3	20	22.7	4	4.5%	12	13.6%	4	4.5%
4	20	22.7	3	3.4%	12	13.6%	5	5.7%
5	66	75.0	19	21.6%	27	30.7%	20	22.7%
6	27	30.7	4	4.5%	16	18.2%	7	7.8%
7	55	62.5	17	19.3%	23	26.1%	15	17.0%
8	18	20.5	6	6.8%	9	10.2%	3	3.4%

Intervention number refers to item under same number in Table 10.
f = frequency   % = per cent of N   N = 88

Section III of the questionnaire contained two parts. The first was a ranking of types of spiritual needs in order of importance to the patient. This data is displayed in Table 9, juxtaposing the modal responses of the Catholic and Protestant subjects. Part 2 requested that the subjects indicate which activities they considered appropriate nursing interventions in the spiritual care area. These data are reported in Tables 10 and 11 within the framework of church affiliation and frequency of church attendance. Both tables point out the two areas most patients see as being legitimate ways to administer spiritual care: "Show kindness, concern, and cheerfulness when giving care," and "Encourage the patient to talk about anything that is bothering him."

Discussion

Interpretation. One of the first findings reported was that, although slightly more than half of the sample were male, more than two-thirds of the subjects verbalizing spiritual needs were female. By chance, one would expect close to 50/50 distribution of spiritual needs according to sex. The Mann-Whitney U statistic also pointed out the difference in responses between men and women. These differences possibly reflect the social conditioning of our culture in which a man may be considered weak if he expresses a need or request for help. He may not be willing to express needs when they are present. It might also mean that because men do not have a socially acceptable avenue for expression of needs they take measures to satisfy their own needs and consequently have less need of help from others. The investigators of the study were female. Perhaps male respondents would have related more openly with a male interviewer. That control variable would be helpful in future studies. The Nurses Christian Fellowship study also reported a reluctance by male subjects to express spiritual needs.

The clergyman was clearly the person preferred by patients for discussing spiritual needs. His role definition and expertise in spiritual concerns suggest the logic to this patient preference. Indeed, the list of the various aspects of spiritual care reveals specific functions that only the clergyman can officially perform. This does not exclude the nurse from providing any spiritual care. Although 40% of respondents believed nurses were not qualified to meet their spiritual needs (Table 7, statement

2), 97% of respondents agreed that nurses give spiritual care by being concerned, cheerful, and kind (statement 4); and 77% agreed that by listening to a patient, a nurse helps them in a spiritual way (statement 10). In the item on ranking of spiritual needs (Table 9), the second most common Protestant response was "expression of caring and support from another person." This is a role that is central to nursing. The largest patient responses to the item on appropriate nursing activities in spiritual care-giving (Table 6) reinforce the concept that listening and concern are types of spiritual care nurses can render.

We may view spiritual care as twofold: specific and technical functions provided exclusively or primarily by the clergyman, and more general, supportive behaviors which can be provided by the layperson as well. The supportive care can be provided by nurses regardless of the religious affiliation of either nurse or patient. The clergy may provide either type of care. The second most important need expressed by Catholic patients was a visit from a clergyman. This may reflect both the need for the specific service of the sacraments (ranked third) and the need for caring in a more general way.

The value of fellowship or caring from another human being is also brought out by the responses to the questions on how the patient felt about the care he received (Table 3) and to what degree his needs were met (Table 4). One respondent commented, "It helped to talk to someone even though it didn't solve my problem." The responses to question 6 of the interview (Table 6) reinforce that a nurse can assist meeting spiritual needs by "nonreligious" behaviors, that is, behaviors not specifically associated with the rituals of particular religions.

Forty-one per cent of the respondents agreed that a patient's beliefs are too personal to discuss with a nurse (Table 7). Does this reflect a lack of confidence in nurses? If nurses were better listeners and rapport between them and their patients greater, would patients respond differently to this question?

The large positive response to the statement that a person who is ill thinks more about his relationship to God may be interpreted to mean that a person's spiritual needs are given more attention during illness than during health (Table 7). Perhaps the illness itself generates more needs. Because often the hospitalized person has an abundance of time and restricted energy and options for physical activities, the opportunity to discover, affirm or alter his philosophy of the meaning of life, illness and death is present. A nurse is in a position to assist a patient when the nurse listens as the patient works through this process. The Mann-Whitney U test (Table 8) showed a significant difference in responses between persons hospitalized only once and those hospitalized 5 or more times in the prior 5 years. This may indicate that repeated hospitalizations, in fact, contribute to a patient's awareness of his spiritual needs.

Frequency of church attendance as an indicator of the degree of interest in spiritual matters was determined to find out if there were differences in the types of spiritual needs experienced and attitudes about spiritual care expressed by the subjects. The findings of this study revealed no significant indications that there are differences, but the scope of the data collection on this area was not sufficient to make any generalizations.

There was a significant z score in measuring the differences in responses between the under-39-years-of-age group and the over-65-years-of-age group. Within the limits of this study, it was not possible to assign cause of difference. It may be that the difference is a function of (1) degree of illness, assuming the older population would have more chronic illness; (2) age alone, assuming a difference in perspective; (3) some other extraneous variable not considered yet. Further study of this question under controlled conditions would be interesting to conduct.

The finding that the sacraments ranked third in importance to Catholic patients (Table 9) is consistent with the findings of the Nurses Christian Fellowship study in which tangible evidence of spiritual value ranked third. In a study by Weiler (Sr. Cashel Weiler, OSF, "Patients' Evaluation of Pastoral Care," *Hospital Progress,* 56 [April 1975] pp. 34-38), the sacraments were first in importance to Catholic patients. The differences in hospitals may account for the difference in the findings. Weiler conducted her study in a Catholic hospital that offered hospital chaplain services so that awareness of the ritual and its importance to patients may have been more prevalent. The present study was conducted in non-denominational private hospitals that offer no structured chaplain services.

In the Nurses Christian Fellowship study 13% of the respondents said that nurses were too busy to help with spiritual needs. This item was included in the current study (Table 7) and agreement was much larger (58%). The reason for so large a difference in this finding may be explained by the instruments used. In the Nurses Christian Fellowship study an interview guide with open-ended questions was used to collect the data. In the present study we used both the interview schedule and a written questionnaire. The item about nurses being too busy was written explicitly for the subject to consider. The presence of the statement made awareness of the patient's feelings overt. Some respondents in the Nurses Christian Fellowship study might have agreed with the statement but did not think about it without a stimulus.

Implications for Nursing. The findings (Table 7) on statement 3 (73% of subjects agreed that a nurse should ask every patient if he or she wishes to see a clergyman) indicate that if this question is not part of an admission procedure or routine nursing care it should be considered. Referral to the clergy is an important part of spiritual care as shown in the ranking of spiritual needs and nurse interventions.

Results of the study indicate that nurses need not feel hesitant to give spiritual care because of being of a different religion than their patients. Since showing kindness and being a sounding board for a patient's ideas were shown to be of great significance, nurses need feel no anxiety if they are not familiar with a patient's theological beliefs. Their responsibility is not to know all the answers but to listen as a patient reviews his beliefs and feelings. They will no doubt learn much over time from listening. The listening function cannot be emphasized strongly enough. Patient responses suggest that the need to talk and to be listened to is not being met.

The area of spiritual care in nursing has not been explored in depth. Studies that explore the relationships of spiritual need to degree of illness, age and sex of patients, and degree of religiosity would be enlightening. When a definite body of knowledge has been developed from these studies, the implications for implementation of the material into nursing education will become apparent.

Limitations. This study was limited in geographical location and in availability of subjects for random sampling. Financial and time constrictions of the investigators narrowed the scope of the study. Time did not permit the pretesting of the questionnaire and data gathered from question 5 were not amenable to analysis. Another weakness of the questionnaire was that there was no place for patient comments other than the structured items except for one "Other" category on one item. The sex of the investigators may have had an inhibiting effect on the responses of the male subjects, and in future studies, it would be helpful to use male interviewers as well as female. Other statistical manipulations by researchers more proficient in statistical methodology might reveal significant findings in the data collected but not thus far realized.

Summary

The purpose of this descriptive study was to determine what spiritual needs hospitalized persons experience, what nursing actions help resolve these needs and how patients feel about receiving spiritual care from a nurse. The convenience sample was composed of noncritical patients from two area general hospitals. Data were collected by using a 34-item questionnaire and an interview guide. The investigators interviewed the subjects after they had completed the questionnaire. Data were subjected to percentage and comparison ratio techniques, and some underwent treatment by the Mann-Whitney U statistic. Findings revealed that females verbalize more spiritual needs than males; that the clergyman is the preferred person with whom patients prefer to speak about spiritual needs; that relief from fear of death, a knowledge of God's presence, expression of caring and support from another person, and receiving the sacraments were ranked the four most important spiritual needs by patients; and that patients appreciate concern and kindness from nurses, and desire to be allowed to talk and to be listened to by nurses.

Awareness and Preparedness of Nurses to Meet Spiritual Needs
Rhonda Chadwick, R.N.

This survey was conducted during 1973 in partial fulfillment of course

Table 12. *Awareness and Preparedness of Nurses to Meet Spiritual Needs*

Question	Choices offered on questionnaire	Per cent*
Do you personally feel that patients have spiritual needs?	yes	100.0
	no	0.0
How long has it been since you last recognized a spiritual need in your patient(s)?	past week	36.4
	past month	39.4
	past six months	9.1
	past year	6.0
	several years ago	0.0
	since beginning career	9.1
	never	0.0
Have you ever read the Bible to or prayed with a patient?	read the Bible to	8.8
	prayed with	29.4
	neither	50.0
	both	11.8
Would you feel comfortable reading the Bible to or praying with a patient?	yes	75.0
	no	3.1
	not sure	21.9
To what degree do you feel that your patients' spiritual needs are met?	completely met	0.0
	well met	6.1
	adequately met	57.6
	poorly met	33.3
	not met at all	3.0
How aware are you as to the religious rites and procedures in the various denominations concerning illness and death? e.g., baptism of a Catholic baby	much knowledge	15.2
	some knowledge	81.8
	little knowledge	3.0
	no knowledge	0.0
Would you like further education in meeting spiritual needs in patients?	yes	60.6
	no	39.4

*A question in which one of the provided answers was not circled or more than one answer was circled was not included in the percentage figure.

requirements in the curriculum of nursing, Delta Junior College, Bay City, Michigan. In a random sample of hospital nurses in the Saginaw, Michigan area representing all three shifts, 34 questionnaires were returned. The results were tabulated into the accompanying table.

The Nurses Christian Fellowship study and the study conducted by Martin, Burrows and Pomilio surveyed patients about their spiritual needs. Chadwick questions nurses and finds a significantly higher percentage of awareness of spiritual needs. She evaluates her findings:

To me, these figures are significant. They indicate that nurses are aware of the presence of spiritual needs in at least some of their patients. 75.0% of the nurses surveyed reported that they would feel comfortable either reading the Bible or praying with a patient. People tend to feel comfortable doing things that carry value to them or are familiar to them. Therefore, I believe that most nurses have had at least some exposure to religious experience.

Yet, why have 50% of them never read the Bible to or prayed with a patient when 75% of them stated they would feel comfortable doing so? I believe that a lack of adequate education in how to apply this willingness greatly accounts for this. I think that because 60.6% of these nurses replied that they would like further education in meeting spiritual needs in patients, there is a need for further education in this area. (Reprinted and adapted from *The Nurses Lamp*, 22, No. 6 [July 1973], pp. 2-3.)

Theses and Dissertations

Nurses writing master's theses or doctoral dissertations about aspects of spiritual care are asked to send a copy to Nurses Christian Fellowship, 6400 Schroeder Rd., P.O. Box 7895, Madison, Wisconsin 53707-7895. Copies of theses or dissertations on file may be ordered from the Nurses Christian Fellowship. Payment of $.10 per page, $5.00 handling charge (per order) and postage costs (1-20 pages $.50; 21-60 pages $1.00; 61-100 pages $1.50, each additional 100 pages $.25) must accompany your order.

Asbury, Linda. "Nurses' Perceptions of Hospitalized Patients' Spiritual Needs Study," 1979, University of Northern Colorado (Undergraduate) 28 pages. ($2.80)

Blecke, Janalou. "Developing a Tool for Determining Appropriate Nurse Action in Meeting Spiritual Needs of Patients in Selected Situations," 1963, University of Washington (Master's thesis) 81 pages. ($8.10)

Chadwick, Rhonda. "Spiritual Needs — How Do They Relate to Patients — How Well Are They Met?" 1972, Delta Junior College (Undergraduate) 10 pages. ($1.00)

Dettmore, Diane. "Nurses' Conceptions and Practices in the Spiritual Dimension of Nursing," 1985, Teachers College, Columbia University (Ph.D. dissertation).*+

Doud, Kim and Travis, Cathy. "The Nurse's Perception of Patients' Spiritual Needs," 1973, University of Iowa (Undergraduate) 44 pages. ($4.40)

Egbert, Emily. "What Is the Relationship between and among Various Indicators of the Quality of Life of Nurses and Their Self-Actualizing Process?" 1982, Walden University (Ph.D. dissertation) 320 total pages (Publication Number LD00544).*+

Fish, Sharon. "Man and His Needs in the Presence of Illness," 1973, University of Rochester (Master's thesis) 93 pages. ($9.30)

Fordyce, Edna. "An Investigation of Television's Potential for Meeting Spiritual Needs of Hospitalized Adult Patients," 1981, Catholic University (Ph.D. dissertation) 193 pages (Publication Number 82-08774).*+

Halstead, Helen. "Self Perceived Well Being among Retired Older Adults: The Positive Side of Aging," 1982, Kansas State University (Ph.D. dissertation) 136 pages. ($13.60)*

Hill, Gay Byington. "Nurse's Description of Institutional Factors Affecting Spiritual Care," 1987, University of Texas-Arlington (Master's thesis) 106 pages. ($10.60)*

Hoskins, Nancy Anness. "Patients' Perceptions of Spiritual Needs," 1986, Vanderbilt University School of Nursing (Master's thesis) 63 pages. ($6.30)*

Hutches, Merilyn, "A Comparison of the Principles of Interpersonal Relationships in Psychiatric Nursing and the Gospels," 1980, California State University-Los Angeles (Master's thesis) 55 pages. ($5.50)

Jones, Ella Rae. "Change of Emphasis in Ministry of Missionary Nurses in Ecuador," 1983, Columbia Graduate School of Bible and Missions (Master's thesis) 193 pages. ($19.30)

Kealey, Carol. "The Patients' Perspective on Spiritual Needs," 1974, University of Missouri-Columbia (Master's thesis) 159 pages. ($15.90)

Lewis, Jean. "A Resource Unit on Spiritual Aspects of Nursing for Basic Nursing Curriculum of a Selected School of Nursing," 1957, University of Washington (Master's thesis) 93 pages. ($9.30)

Lowe, Ann Sherry. "God as an Intimate Confidant," 1979, California State University-Long Beach (Master's thesis) 74 pages. ($7.40)*

Martin, Claire. "Spiritual Needs of Patients," 1971, State University of New York-Utica-Rome (Undergraduate) 41 pages. ($4.10)

Nelson, Barbara. "A Survey: How Graduate Nurses in Maternal Child Health Perceive Their Role in the Spiritual Dimension of Nursing Care," 1976, Boston University (Master's thesis) 113 pages. ($11.30)

Nelson, Barbara E. "Preparation for Ministry within the Context of Nursing: Clinical Pastoral Education," 1983, Andover Newton Theological School (Ph.D. dissertation) 178 pages. ($17.80)*

Phinney, Richard P. "Study of the Characteristics of Spiritual

Experiences of the Older Adult Using a Phenomenological Approach," 1986, Gwynedd-Mercy College (Master's thesis) 106 pages. ($10.60)*

Piles, Carole. "Spiritual Care as Part of the Nursing Curriculum — A Descriptive Study," 1980, St. Louis University (Master's thesis) 91 pages. ($9.10)*

Piles, Carole. "Spiritual Care: Role of Nursing Education and Practice — A Needs Survey for Curriculum Development," 1986, St. Louis University (Ph.D. dissertation) 196 pages. ($19.60)*

Schomus, Irene G. "Hospital Stress and the Patient's Perception of the Importance of Spiritual Needs," 1980, Arizona State University (Master's thesis) 123 pages. ($12.30)*

Simsen, Barbara. "Spiritual Needs and Resources in Illness and Hospitalization," 1985, University of Manchester (England) (Master's thesis) 450 pages. ($45.00)*

Slaughter, Terry Ann. "Identifying the Spiritual Needs of the Oncology Patient," 1979, University of Arizona (Master's thesis) 71 pages. ($7.10)*

Stallwood, Jean and Flor, Eleanor. "Spiritual Needs — What Do Patients Say?" 1970 (for NCF) 11 pages. ($1.10)

Stoll, Ruth. "Indicators of Life Satisfaction in Persons with Life Threatening Diagnosis and Those with a Non-Life Threatening Diagnosis," 1983, Catholic University of America (Ph.D. dissertation). +

Strasser, Judith A. "The Relation of General Forgiveness and Forgiveness Type to Reported Health in the Elderly," 1984, Catholic University of America (Ph.D. dissertation) 197 pages (Publication Number 84-16059).* +

Swanborg, Nancy K. "Holistic Health Care: Ministry to the Health Care Professional," 1984, Marygrove College (Master's thesis) 59 pages. ($5.90)

Thompson, Arlene and McDough, Carolyn. "Manual on Spiritual Needs with Focus on the Obstetric Patient," 1968 or 69, Ohio State University (project) 57 pages. ($5.70)

Thompson, Mary. "An Investigation of the Relationship of Love, Mutuality, Freedom and Newness with the Perception of Hope in

Patients with the Diagnosis of Cancer," 1980, California State-Los Angeles (Master's thesis) 164 pages. ($16.40)

Tripp, Kathleen. "The Relationship between Stress and Importance of Spiritual Needs Among Ambulatory Care Clients," 1979, Arizona State University (Master's thesis) 137 pages. ($13.70)*

Walker, Virginia. "Spiritual Needs of Adolescents Who Seek Primary Health Care," 1982, University of Rochester-Rochester, NY (Master's thesis) 109 pages. ($10.90)*

Williams, Eleanor. "A Spiritual Needs Assessment Tool," 1985, California State University-Long Beach (Master's thesis) 107 pages. ($10.70)*

Yanosh, Norann. "Patients Perception of Spiritual Needs and Concomitant Nurse Action," 1966, Ohio State University (Master's thesis) 78 pages. ($7.80)

* Indicates Abstract available.
+ Indicates the dissertation is copyrighted and should be ordered from the University Microfilms International, Dissertation Copies, P.O. Box 1764, Ann Arbor, MI 48106 (include publication number when listed).

Appendix B
Nurses Christian Fellowship

Nursing sprang from the roots of Christian faith and has traditionally been a caring vocation. Today nursing is in a state of change and transition. Nurses are seeking new values and ethical standards. They are developing changing philosophies of caring based on those beliefs and values. In this era of uncertainty, NCF seeks to re-establish a Christian philosophy of nursing. Our concern is for quality nursing care which includes the spiritual dimension and reflects the gospel of Jesus Christ. We aim to encourage nurses and nursing students to become increasingly aware of their potential as Christians in the practice of nursing, and to recognize their responsibilities for active participation in the nursing profession.

Nurses Christian Fellowship began in Chicago in the mid 1930s when three nurses began meeting to pray at Children's Hospital. The group grew and spread across the country. In 1948 NCF became a national organization. The three stated purposes of NCF groups are (1) to assist nurses and nursing students to witness to Jesus Christ as Lord and Savior within the nursing milieu, (2) to help nurses and nursing students to grow in Christian maturity and apply the Christian faith to nursing practice, and (3) to encourage nurses to find God's place for them in the worldwide mission of the church.

Today Nurses Christian Fellowship chapters can be found in more than one hundred schools of nursing. Another one hundred groups of nurses meet in hospitals, health agencies and metropolitan areas. NCF staff serve these groups by providing leadership training, assistance with program planning, resource material and general encouragement. Groups study the Bible, pray together, discuss problems and issues they confront in nursing, and encourage and support one another in day-by-day Christian living. Some sponsor areawide workshops relating faith and nursing.

The NCF national organization provides a number of resources to assist individuals and groups. *The Nurse's Role in Spiritual Care* workshop is designed to prepare nurses to meet the spiritual needs of patients. *Christian Discipleship in Nursing,* NCF's summer conferences, are one-week institutes giving students and nurses in-depth exposure to a portion of Scripture, the spiritual dimension of nursing, and caring relationships. Conferences and workshops often grant continuing education credit. *Love That Heals* seminars train nurses and laypersons to visit the ill and lonely in their churches.

Literature provided by NCF is another important resource for nurses and nursing students. *Caring in Crisis* (InterVarsity Press) is a Bible study guide providing the biblical basis for *Spiritual Care: The Nurse's Role. The Spiritual Needs of Children* (IVP) describes the unique spiritual needs of children from a growth and development perspective. *Spiritual Dimensions of Mental Health* deals with the relationship between Christianity and psychiatric/mental health nursing. *Not Just a Job* (IVP) offers a biblical perspective on work and applies that perspective to practical issues related to time, money, and marriage and the church. *Missionary Nurse Survey* assists nurses preparing for missionary service. Bible study guides (listed in Appendix C) apply biblical principles to everyday experiences in nursing. Publication of the quarterly *Journal of Christian Nursing* began in 1984.

The *Journal of Christian Nursing* features professional articles on topics like these: spiritual care, ethical issues, crosscultural nursing, nurses' and patients' experiences. The magazine maintains a lively, personal, readable style. For subscription information write *Journal of Christian Nursing,* P.O. Box 1650, Downers Grove, IL 60515.

Officially, Nurses Christian Fellowship is a department of InterVarsity Christian Fellowship (IVCF) which is incorporated in the State of Illinois as a nonprofit religious corporation. NCF is represented on IVCF's Board by nurses who are active in the profession. They, together with NCF staff, assist the Director and Staff Directors in formulating the program. NCF is represented regularly with an exhibit, and frequently with program offerings, at the American Nurses Association Conventions, National League for Nursing Conventions, National Student Nurses Association Conventions and various state conventions.

Nurses Christian Fellowship has no guaranteed income. We are dependent on the gifts and prayers of concerned Christians to meet our budget.

For more information, write to Nurses Christian Fellowship, 6400 Schroeder Road, P.O. Box 7895, Madison, Wisconsin 53707-7895.

Appendix C
Study Guides for Nurses

From InterVarsity Press

Dilemma: A Nurse's Guide for Making Ethical Decisions. Judith Allen Shelly presents a clear, comprehensive procedure for thinking through ethical dilemmas in the light of Scripture. Includes eight clinical case studies to help readers turn theory into practice. paper, 168 pages

Caring in Crisis: Bible Studies for Helping People. Judith Allen Shelly offers six weeks of individual studies with a group study for each week to help Christians understand their responsibility to meet the spiritual needs of people. paper, 36 daily studies; 6 weekly discussions

Lifestyle of Love. These studies from John 13—17 focus on Christ and his example for us as nurses. We see him as our role model—helping people in crisis, praying, identifying priorities. paper, 8 studies

Rough Edges of the Christian Life. Here are topical studies particularly appropriate for beginning nursing students. Titles include "Who Am I?" "Confidence," "Love," "Fear" and "Anxiety." These studies may be used either in individual or group study. paper, 8 studies

From Nurse's Christian Fellowship

Following the Great Physician. Six studies from the Gospels designed to identify principles taught and demonstrated by Jesus Christ for relating with people. The studies are excellent for R.N.'s, experienced students and others with patient contacts. Topics include "Offering Peace to People Facing Death," "Communicating Forgiveness" and "Comforting Relatives Experiencing Grief."

Provided We Suffer. One purpose of these studies is to provide a balanced biblical view of suffering and healing. Subjects include "Caring for Those Who Suffer," "Suffering: Used by God" and "Healing: Our Involvement." These studies are best used after *Following the Great Physician.*

Living in Hope. Hope is like love—a feeling, hard to pinpoint; a concept. But more than that, hope is seen in actions which reflect what is inside a person. This series of eight studies includes such topics as "Our Living Hope," "Hope—Where Do You Find It?" "Hope—Based on the Character of God" and "Grieve, But with Hope."

Walking through the Valley. This series of studies helps us look at the scriptural perspective of death and dying. One objective for the studies is to help nurses learn to communicate God's love and care to those facing death as well as to their families.

A Lifestyle of Joy. Seven studies from Philippians which focus on seeing how we can reflect Jesus Christ in nursing. Studies include "Joy in Serving," "Rejoicing in the Lord," "Christ-Centered Goals" and "Joy in Living and Dying."

God's Provision for Human Needs. Eight studies focusing on God's provision for psychological needs, for safety and security, for love, the feeling of belonging and self-esteem.

Mental Health: A Biblical Perspective. Eight studies looking at some of the aspects of a definition of mental health: "A state of dynamic equilibrium characterized by hope, love, joy, peace where relationships with God, self, others and the world around are mediated by the love of God and wherein one experiences the peace of God about the past, present and future."

Studies in Assertiveness. This is a popular and controversial subject today, but what does Scripture say? These six studies look at models for, motives for and methods of assertiveness.

Colossian Capsules. Twenty brief studies which cover the entire letter to the Colossians. Appropriate for personal or small group Bible study. Looks at "Establishing a Christian Identity," "Christian Living in the World," "Preparing for Ministry" and "Doing the Work."

Forgiveness and Reconciliation. Six studies designed to assist in growing in forgiveness and understanding. Studies include "Living as Forgiving People" and "Restored to Love."

Radical Christian Living in a Secular World. Six studies from the Sermon on the Mount (Mt 5—7) designed to help us be Christ's people who live as Christ's people in our world. Includes "Radical Purity," "Radical Peace" and "Radical Obedience."

A complete list of study materials with prices is available from Nurses Christian Fellowship, 6400 Schroeder Road, P.O. Box 7895, Madison, Wisconsin 53707-7895. Send a stamped, self-addressed envelope with your request for the list.

Notes

Chapter 1
[1]*Christianity Today,* 27 Aug. 1976, p. 35.
[2]An excellent discussion of varying concepts of God can be found in J.B. Phillips, *Your God Is Too Small* (New York: Macmillan, 1974).
[3]See the rest of Paul's speech in Acts 17:16-31.
[4]Samuel Southard, *Religion and Nursing* (Nashville: Broadman Press, 1959), p. 54.
[5]Ruth Lichtenberger, "The Patients' Right to Spiritual Care," *Transfusions,* Mar. 1977, pp. 1-2.
[6]"1973 Code for Nurses," *American Journal of Nursing,* 73, Aug. 1973, p. 1351.
[7]Laurence Urdang, ed., *The Random House Dictionary of the English Language, College Edition* (New York: Random House, 1969).
[8]Imogene M. King, *Toward a Theory for Nursing* (New York: John Wiley and Sons, 1971), p. 72.

Chapter 2
[1]Hans Walter Wolff, *Anthropology of the Old Testament* (Philadelphia: Fortress Press, 1975, p. 107. See also Psalm 88:10-12; 115:17; Isaiah 38:18.
[2]Ibid., p. 111.
[3]See 1 John 3:14; 4:7, 19.
[4]For a fuller description of secular society see Alvin Toffler, *Future Shock* (New York: Bantam Books, 1970).
[5]See Romans 1:18-32; 2:15.
[6]For an extensive treatment of the problem of guilt, see Paul Tournier, *Guilt and Grace,* trans. Arthur Heatcote (New York: Harper & Row, 1962).
[7]The importance of meaning and purpose in life is discussed in Viktor Frankl, *Man's Search for Meaning,* trans. Ilse Lasch (New York: Washington Square Press, 1971).
[8]See Ephesians 2:1-3; Galatians 5:19-21; Colossians 2:8; 3:5-11.
[9]See 1 Thessalonians 3:1-8; 2 Corinthians 1:3-7.
[10]See Hebrews 2.
[11]Vernon Grounds, "God's Perspective on Man," *Journal of the American Scientific Affiliation,* 28 Dec. 1976, 146.
[12]Wolff, p. 62.
[13]Ibid., p. 10.
[14]Ibid., p. 28.
[15]Henry Chadwick, *The Early Church* (Grand Rapids: Eerdmans, 1968), p. 34.

Chapter 3
[1]Sister Mary Hubert, "Spiritual Care for Every Patient," *The Journal of Nursing Education,* May-June 1963, p. 11.
[2]Paul Steeves, *Getting to Know God* (Downers Grove, Ill.: InterVarsity Press, 1973), p. 94.

[3]Luke 15:11-32.

[4]Jean Stallwood, "Spiritual Dimensions of Nursing Practice" in *Clinical Nursing*, ed. Irene Beland and Joyce Passos, 3rd ed. (New York: Macmillan, 1975), p. 1088.

[5]Joyce Travelbee, *Interpersonal Aspects of Nursing*, Edition 2 (Philadelphia: F. A. Davis, 1971), p. 16.

[6]See Viktor E. Frankl, *Man's Search for Meaning* (New York: Washington Square Press, 1971), and Viktor E. Frankl, *The Doctor and the Soul* (New York: Alfred A. Knopf, 1972), for a discussion of the theory of logotherapy or existential analysis which focuses on the human search for a higher meaning in life.

[7]Viktor E. Frankl, *Man's Search for Meaning*, p. xiii.

[8]Viktor E. Frankl, *The Doctor and the Soul*, p. xv.

[9]See Job 1—42 for a complete account. A highly readable translation is found in the Good News Bible, Today's English Version. The book of Job is available separately in this version as *Tried and True: Job for Modern Man*, (New York: American Bible Society, 1971). Chapters 1—2 focus on the events that precipitated Job's crisis; chapters 3—37 describe Job's response to the crisis; chapters 38—42 discuss God's answer to Job's questions. For a poetic account of Job see Thomas John Carlisle, *Journey with Job* (Grand Rapids: Eerdmans, 1976).

[10]William E. Hulme, *Dialogue in Despair* (Nashville, Abingdon Press, 1968), p. 146. A helpful commentary on Job.

[11]Ibid., p. 146.

[12]From Judy VanHeukelem, "Thoughts on Hope," *The Nurses Lamp*, 26, No. 5, (May 1975).

[13]Isaiah 53 speaks of the coming Messiah who will make people whole; Micah 5:2-4 prophesies the birth of the Messiah; Malachi 3:1-4 looks to the Messiah who will refine and purify Israel.

[14]Acts 28:20 says Jesus is the hope of Israel; Matthew 12:21 and Romans 15:12 say Jesus is also the hope of the Gentiles (Isaiah 42:1-4 and Isaiah 11:10); 1 Thessalonians 1:3 and 1:10 tell the people to hope in the Lord Jesus Christ who is a deliverer; Titus 2:13 says to hope in the great God and Savior Jesus Christ.

[15]New Testament passages dealing with Jesus as the person who bridges the gap between human beings and God are John 3:1-21; 6:22-59; 14:1-7; 17:1-3.

[16]Ashley Montagu, *Touching: The Human Significance of the Skin* (New York: Columbia Univ. Press, 1971), pp. 82-84.

[17]Masumi Toyotome, *Three Kinds of Love* (Downers Grove, Ill.: InterVarsity Press, 1961). Nursing implications in this section are drawn from Toyotome's analysis of the varying kinds of love.

[18]Ibid., pp. 8-9.

[19]Feelings related to a lack or supply of love and relatedness were identified by a group of nurses at a conference sponsored by Nurses Christian Fellowship, "The Role of the Nurse in Spiritual Care," March 18-19, 1977, Liberty Corner, New Jersey.

[20]A. W. Tozer, *The Knowledge of the Holy* (New York: Harper & Row, 1961), pp. 105-06.

[21]Karl Menninger, *Whatever Became of Sin?* (New York: Hawthorn Books, 1973), pp. 1-2.

[22]Tournier, p. 10.

[23]See Isaiah 53:6; Romans 3:23.

[24]Robert M. Horn, *Go Free!* (Downers Grove, Ill.: InterVarsity Press, 1976), p. 16.

[25]"The Role of the Nurse in Spiritual Care" Conference.

[26]Peter S. Ford, *The Healing Trinity* (New York: Harper & Row, 1971), pp. 1-6.

[27]G. Keith Parker, "Pastoral Care of Chronically Ill Patients," in *Pastoral Care in Crucial Human Situations*, ed. Wayne E. Oates and Andrew D. Lester (Valley Forge: Judson Press, 1969), pp. 178-79.

[28]Horn, p. 44.

[29]See Isaiah 53; John 3:16-21; Romans 5.
[30]See Isaiah 55:7; Acts 16:30-31.
[31]See John 1:12; Romans 8:22-23; Ephesians 1:3-10.
[32]See Luke 7:48-50; Romans 5:1-5; John 16:33; John 14.
[33]See 1 John 1:9.

Chapter 4

[1]Travelbee, pp. 16, 65, 170, 175. Beland and Passos, pp. 13, 1086.
[2]Travelbee, p. 159.
[3]Martin J. Heinecken, *Christian Teachings* (Philadelphia: Fortress Press, 1967), p. 223.
[4]A similar interview guide, developed for Nurses Christian Fellowship by Ruth Stoll, Louisville, Kentucky, in 1971, served as the basis for this guide.
[5]For an example of a nursing history format which includes the spiritual dimension, see Beland, p. 29.
[6]Mi Ja Kim and Derry Ann Moritz, *Classification of Nursing Diagnoses: Proceedings of the Third and Fourth National Conferences* (New York: McGraw-Hill, 1982), p. 219.
[7]Ibid., p. 242.
[8]Margaret Lunney, "Nursing Diagnosis: Refining the System," *American Journal of Nursing 82* (March 1982):456.
[9]Kim and Moritz, *Classification*, p. 388.
[10]Ibid., p. 332.
[11]Judith Allen Shelly et al., *The Spiritual Needs of Children* (Downers Grove, Ill.: Inter-Varsity Press, 1982), pp. 138-40.
[12]Kim and Moritz, *Classification*, p. 315.
[13]Ibid., p. 314.
[14]Judith Van Heukelem in Shelly, *Spiritual Needs*, pp. 94-95.

Chapter 5

[1]Travelbee, p. 19.
[2]Bonnie J. Meyer, R.N., unpublished manuscript.
[3]For a further expansion on listening and communication see Reuel L. Howe, *The Miracle of Dialogue* (New York: Seabury Press, 1963).
[4]For example, Dosia Carlson, *The Unbroken Vigil* (Richmond: John Knox Press, 1968); Joni Eareckson, with Joe Musser, *Joni* (Minneapolis: World Wide Publications, 1976); Joseph Bayly, *The View from a Hearse* (Elgin, Ill.: David C. Cook, 1970).
[5]See Gary R. Collins, "Burn Out: The Hazard of Professional People Helpers," *Christianity Today*, 1 Apr. 1977, pp. 12-14.
[6]Gabriel Marcel, *The Philosophy of Existence*, trans. Manya Harari (New York: Philosophical Library, 1949), p. 26.
[7]From the diary of Sharon Fish, R.N.
[8]Romans 12:15-16.
[9]Sister Madeleine Clemence, "Existentialism: A Philosophy of Commitment," *American Journal of Nursing*, 66 (Mar. 1966), 504.

Chapter 6

[1]Henri J. M. Nouwen, *Intimacy* (Notre Dame: Fides Publishers, 1969), p. 75.
[2]Daniel C. DeArment, "Prayer and the Dying Patient: A Way of Intimacy Without Exposure," *Princeton Seminary Bulletin*, 66, No. 2 (Summer 1974), p. 55.
[3]Travelbee, p. 16.
[4]DeArment, p. 56.
[5]See Luke 8:48; 18:42.
[6]See 2 Corinthians 12:8-9; 1 Timothy 5:23; 2 Timothy 4:20.

Chapter 7

[1]See 2 Timothy 3:16; 2 Peter 1:10-21.
[2]See John 20:30-31; Romans 15:4-6.

³See Psalm 103.
⁴See Luke 2:11; Acts 13:23; Ephesians 1:7; 1 John 4:14.
⁵See Psalm 23; John 10:1-18; Hebrews 13:20.
⁶See 1 Corinthians 12:4-11; Romans 12:3-8; 1 Peter 4:10-11.
⁷Paul Tournier, *A Doctor's Casebook in the Light of the Bible,* trans. Edwin Hudson (London: SCM Press, 1969), p. 22.
⁸Bayly, pp. 40-41.
⁹From Alice Caldwell, "A Nurse's Climb," *The Nurses Lamp,* 27, No. 1 (Sept. 1975).
¹⁰Hulme, pp. 20-21.
¹¹A resource for the use of Scripture in pastoral counseling is Wayne E. Oates, *The Bible in Pastoral Care* (Grand Rapids: Baker Book House, 1973).
¹²Eareckson, pp. 48-49.

Chapter 8
¹Mary Risley, *The House of Healing* (New York: Doubleday, 1961), p. 203.
²Rev. Larry VandeCreek, Th.M., and Jerry Royer, M.D., "Education for Interdisciplinary Teamwork," *Journal of Pastoral Care,* 29, No. 3 (Sept. 1975), p. 182.
³Howard J. Clinebell, in *Healing and Wholeness,* ed. D. Wayne Montgomery (Richmond: John Knox Press, 1971), p. 15.
⁴For further elaboration see Beland and Passos, pp. 4-5; and the *Journal of Pastoral Care,* Dec. 1976, pp. 217-21.
⁵Beland and Passos, p. 11.
⁶This quote is from the Augsburg Confession of the Lutheran Church. Other Christian denominations have similar statements. See *The Common Catechism,* ed. Johannes Feiner and Lukas Vischer (New York: Seabury, 1975), pp. 676-81.

Chapter 9
¹Collins, pp. 12-14.
²Roberta Lyder, "The Quest," *The Nurses Lamp,* Mar. 1973, pp. 1-2.
³From the personal diary of Bonnie J. Meyer, R.N.
⁴Adapted from Judy Allen, "Getting Started: A Graduate Group," *The Nurses Lamp,* Sept. 1974, pp. 3-4.

Scripture Index

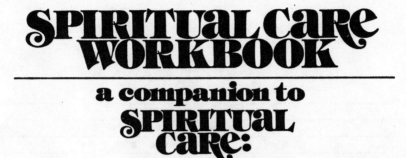

SPIRITUAL CARE WORKBOOK

a companion to SPIRITUAL CARE:
The Nurse's Role

Judith Allen Shelly
R.N., B.S.N., M.A.R.

INTERVARSITY PRESS
DOWNERS GROVE, ILLINOIS 60515

Introduction

The purpose of this workbook is to help you apply the principles in the textbook, *Spiritual Care: The Nurse's Role*, to nursing situations and your own life. Nursing is an applied science and a practical art. Nursing theory is useful only if it constructively affects patient care. If the spiritual dimension of nursing remains only an interesting idea, it is of no value. This workbook is designed for nurses who want to translate theory into responsible actions that will help meet the spiritual needs of patients in concrete ways.

Who Should Use This Workbook? This workbook is designed for several groups. For *nursing faculty*, material in the text and workbook is arranged to provide the basis for a semester course on the spiritual dimension of nursing. The material can also be integrated into existing curricula. *Nurses and nursing students* may want to use the text and workbook as an independent study project. For *student and graduate fellowships*, the text and workbook can provide the basis for weekly or monthly Nurses Christian Fellowship meetings. The material is also readily adaptable to *in-service or continuing education courses* in health-care facilities. Finally, it is our hope that this workbook and the text are adaptable to a wide variety of *health-care workers*, other than nurses, to *physicians*, to *hospital chaplains*, to *ministers* who visit hospitals and to all *those with visitation ministries*.

The Workbook Format This workbook consists of nine two-part units. One or more chapters of the *Spiritual Care* text serves as prerequisite reading for each unit except unit eight. Each unit is introduced by objectives and a self-study exercise requiring one to three hours to complete. The independent work provides the basis for a small group session which concludes each unit. Small group sessions are designed to be completed in one hour though they can easily be expanded to ninety minutes. Note that a tenth small group is possible by extending session seven.

Guidelines for Small Groups Small group sessions are designed for groups of four to eight members. If you have more than eight people, break into smaller sections. It will be helpful to have an even number in each group since session five will be done in pairs. Group dynamics will be facilitated if group membership is stable and attendance regular. Both content and interpersonal relationships build on the foundation laid in previous sessions; therefore, the sessions should be covered in the order listed. No sessions should be omitted. Each week one person should be responsible for guiding the group through the exercise. This will facilitate group interaction and help develop leadership skills. Instructions are built into each small group session. They include an introduction, directions for use of special materials and discussion questions.

If You Are a Course Leader or Small Group Leader The chart on page 8 gives a course outline with objectives for each unit. Note that in most instances some advance preparation by the course leader or group leader is necessary. Special materials are needed for units two, three, four and eight. These materials can be ordered before the course begins. A checklist of materials, equipment and arrangements necessary for each small group session is provided on page 9 to facilitate organization. All materials should be ordered *at least six weeks in advance* of the date you need them. Each person should have a copy of both the text and workbook.

At the end of this course of study you should be able to recognize basic spiritual needs of patients and intervene responsibly by utilizing the steps of the nursing process. My prayer is that you will find the spiritual dimension of nursing personally fulfilling and professionally rewarding.

Course Outline and Objectives

Unit	1 Responsible Nursing	2 What Is Man?	3 What Are Spiritual Needs?	4 Spiritual Needs and the Nursing Process
Prerequisite Reading	Text: Chapter 1	Text: Chapter 2	Text: Chapter 3	Text: Chapter 4
Individual Objectives	To recognize the mandate for spiritual care within the context of professional nursing.	To explore personal and biblical views of man as a foundation for spiritual care.	To identify spiritual needs in yourself and others.	To enter into the nursing process from the spiritual aspect in four nursing situations.
Group Objectives	That the group members will: 1. express personal convictions about spiritual care; 2. demonstrate their present level of expertise to the group; and 3. recognize their mandate to provide spiritual care.	That the group members will: 1. demonstrate an understanding of the biblical view of man; and 2. express their personal identities within the group.	That the group members will: 1. be able to define a spiritual need; 2. observe patients by role-plays and identify their spiritual needs; and 3. discuss clues to the patient's spiritual needs and describe how each is related to a relationship with God or lack thereof.	That the group members will: 1. observe and interpret spiritual needs of four role-played patients; 2. plan nursing invention based on above; and 3. evaluate the care planned and respond to comments in part C of case studies.

★　＊

5 Use of Self/ Use of Prayer	6 Use of Scripture/Referral to Clergy	7 Utilizing Our Resources	7a Resources Continued (optional)	8 Putting It all Together	9 Personal Resources/Evaluating
Text: Chapters 5 & 6	Text: Chapters 7 & 8	Review Text: Chapters 3—8		Job (Today's English Version)	Text: Chapter 9
To explore what you have to offer a patient by the therapeutic use of self and to communicate with God about your own needs and the needs of patients.	To explore the resources of Scripture for personal and professional use and to discover what resources are available through the hospital chaplain.	To analyze your ability to utilize the principles of spiritual care with a patient.	To give you more time to prepare additional verbatims.	To review and apply your knowledge of spiritual needs, the nursing process and the use of nursing resources for spiritual care using the book of Job as a case study.	To explore your personal spiritual resources and make plans to utilize them more fully.
That the group members will: 1. practice the use of self and prayer with another student; 2. evaluate each other's performance in listening and empathy; and 3. experience the vulnerability and commitment that develop when spiritual needs are discussed and met.	That the group members will: 1. share their past experiences with Scripture with the group; and 2. understand how the hospital chaplain views himself as a resource to patients and nurses.	That the group members will: 1. evaluate their ability to utilize nursing resources for spiritual care; and 2. discuss verbatims so as to support and encourage the presenters and learn from their successes and difficulties.	That each member will have the opportunity to present a verbatim to the group; sessions may be added at this point.	That the group members will evaluate how well they have applied concepts and principles presented in this course.	That the group members will: 1. discuss and evaluate their personal support systems; 2. evaluate the meaningfulness and usefulness of the group to them personally and professionally; and 3. determine whether to continue the group.

✓　　★　　＊　★　　★

KEY ＊ special materials needed ★ advance preparation by group leader required ✓ done in pairs

Advance Planning Sheet for Group Leaders

Unit	Date	Preparations Necessary
1		☐ Chalkboard or other visual aid
2		☐ 8½ x 11 white paper for each group member ☐ Crayons or colored markers
6		☐ Ask hospital chaplain to attend session and give him a copy of questions he will be asked ☐ Chalkboard or other visual aid
7		☐ Copies of verbatims to be presented
8		☐ Order "Tried and True" (Job in the Today's English Version) from the American Bible Society for each participant, P.O. Box 5656, Grand Central Station, N.Y., NY 10017. ☐ Chalkboard or other visual aid
9		☐ (optional) Order samples of small group Bible study guides as follow-up tools. (See appendix C of text.)

Unit 1
Responsible Nursing
Individual Exercise
Prerequisite reading: Chapter one, *Spiritual Care: The Nurse's Role*

Is spiritual care a necessary part of responsible nursing? If we believe that human beings are created by God and that the need for a relationship with God is fundamental to a person's nature, then we will recognize that this need becomes our primary mandate to give spiritual care. Spiritual care promotes health and contributes to the well-being of the whole person. The objective for unit one is to enable you to recognize the mandate for spiritual care within the context of professional nursing as well as to evaluate your own involvement with patients spiritually.

To know what responsible nursing is, we must first define nursing.

1/Look up the definition of nursing in at least two current nursing texts (preferably texts used in your school of nursing curriculum).

Text _____

Definition _____

Text _____

Definition _____

(optional) You might want to compare these definitions with the ideas of our "foremother" in nursing. Most libraries will have Florence Nightingale's *Notes on Nursing* (New York: Appleton and Company, 1860). It is delightful reading!

(optional) In most states you will receive a copy of the state's "Nurse Practice Act" with your professional license. In it you will find the legal definition of nursing in your state. Compare this definition with those you have found in nursing texts.

2/How would *you* define nursing?

3/Do the definitions of nursing you have listed restrict you in any way from meeting spiritual needs?

4/In what ways do the definitions give you a mandate for meeting spiritual needs of patients?

5/Have you ever attempted to meet a patient's spiritual needs? If you have, write a brief description of your most recent attempt. Include (a) how you assessed the spiritual need, (b) your intervention and rationale, and (c) the patient's response.

Note: Be sure to bring your workbook with you to small group sessions.

Small Group Session

T hroughout history, nursing has recognized human beings as spiritual beings with spiritual needs; many of us, however, have been taught that religion is a controversial subject we should avoid discussing with patients. Nurses may feel uncomfortable about meeting spiritual needs. This first small group session provides an opportunity for people to share thoughts, feelings, fears, reservations, expectations and experiences. The overall purpose of the session is to set the tone for the remaining group sessions and establish a climate of support and encouragement.

If group members do not know each other, spend a few minutes on introductions. You may also want to take a few minutes to share what each person hopes to learn from the course. Then focus on these items:

1/Discussion questions.

a/Do you think patients have a right to spiritual care? Why or why not? (10 minutes)

b/Do you feel you have a right or a responsibility as a nurse to provide spiritual care? (10 minutes)

2/Share experiences group members have had in meeting spiritual needs of patients. People can share the examples they wrote about in question 5 of the individual exercise. (30 minutes)

Leader's Notes
Remind group members to bring their workbook to all small group sessions.
Independent work is the basis for many small group discussion questions.

Unit 2
What Is Man?
Individual Exercise
Prerequisite reading: Chapter two, *Spiritual Care: The Nurse's Role*

Who am I?" is one of the most frequently asked questions today. Most people seem unsure of the answer. Our perceptions of who we are depend to a large extent on our conceptual model of man. That model also forms the basis for the nursing care we give. The objective for unit two is to enable you to explore personal and biblical views of man as a foundation for giving spiritual care.

1/*Who are you?* If you wanted someone to know the "real you," how would you describe yourself?

2/In what ways do your relationships with other people define who you are?

3/What gives your life meaning and purpose?

4/Do you like yourself? Why or why not?

5/What things would you like to change about yourself?

6/Several people in the Old Testament wondered about their identities. Look up these passages and write down how each of the people found their identity defined. What primary relationship was involved? Exodus 3:11, 12

Jeremiah 1:4-8

Psalm 8:3-8

Psalm 139:1-18

7/In what ways does your relationship with God establish who you are?

8/*Man is a physically, psychosocially and spiritually integrated being, created to live in harmony with God, himself and others.* To get a full grasp of our working concept of man, look up these words in a dictionary and write down a definition for each one:
integrated—

created—

harmony—

9/What does it mean for *you* to be in harmony with yourself?

with others?

with God?

10/What *factors* help you establish and maintain harmony with yourself?

with others?

with God?

Small Group Session

T his session will help your group think through how a particular view of, or beliefs about, human nature affect nursing practice. The group members will also take a look at themselves and begin to share their uniqueness with each other. The question "What is man?" becomes meaningful to us personally when it is asked more specifically: "Who am I?" and "Who are you?"

What Is Man? (30 minutes) Discuss these questions based on chapter two of the text:
1/What effect should the knowledge that your patient is created by God and for God have on your nursing care?

2/Genesis 1:26 says that we are created in God's image. What does that mean? In what ways should your nursing care be influenced by this knowledge?

3/The biblical view is that each person is an integrated whole. This differs from a dualistic view common to Greek philosophy as well as to most Eastern religions. Here are summarizations of dualistic views. Discuss the implications each of these could have on nursing care if held by a patient or a nurse.
a/The body is irrelevant or evil; only the soul, or spirit, is good.

b/Each person contains a "spark of divinity" (the spirit or soul) which seeks to be free from the body that entraps it to merge with an impersonal supreme being or energy force.

Who Are You? (30 minutes) When we are secure in our own identity, we can begin to appreciate and respect the uniqueness of others. We can also enjoy our common humanity. After making paper and colored pens available, have group members spend 10 minutes writing the answers to questions 4-8. Then discuss question 9 for the remaining 20 minutes of the session.
4/In the center of your paper draw a stick figure to represent yourself. Use a color that represents how you feel about yourself in general.

5/Draw a circle around the stick figure to represent your world in a color that expresses how you feel about life.

6/Draw stick figures to represent each of the most significant people in your life (past and present) in colors that express how you feel about each of them.

7/Above the stick figure representing yourself draw symbols to represent your main goals in life.

8/Below the stick figure representing yourself draw symbols for the things which give your life meaning and purpose.

9/Share your drawings with the group and explain the significance of your symbols.

Unit 3
What Are Spiritual Needs?
Individual Exercise
Prerequisite reading: Chapter three, *Spiritual Care: The Nurse's Role*

T he objective for this unit is to enable you to identify spiritual needs in yourself and others. *A spiritual need is the lack of any factor or factors necessary to establish and/or maintain a dynamic, personal relationship with God.*

Among the factors necessary to establish and maintain a dynamic, personal relationship with God are (1) meaning and purpose, (2) love and relatedness, and (3) forgiveness. We begin to meet our patients' spiritual needs by understanding our own needs and how they are met.

Meaning and Purpose

1/What are you living for?

2/What has been the primary influence in shaping your life goals?

3/Would the loss of any body part or function affect your meaning and purpose in life? Which one(s)? How?

4/Would the loss of any relationship alter your meaning and purpose in life? Which one(s)? How?

5/What does death mean to you?

Love and Relatedness

6/List your most significant relationships. Give reasons why each of these is important to you.

7/Where and with whom do you feel the most loved?

8/What are some of the ways you perceive that someone loves and cares about you?

9/What makes you feel insecure about another person's love for you?

10/Do you feel God loves you? What factors have made you feel as you do?

Forgiveness

11/When you feel bitterness and resentment toward someone, how does this affect your overall attitude toward life?

12/What effect do guilt feelings have on you?

13/How do you handle your feelings of guilt, anger, resentment and bitterness?

14/How do you experience forgiveness from a human friend?

15/How do you experience forgiveness from God?

Summary of Your Spiritual Needs
16/Using the definition of spiritual needs and the self-assessment you have made (include data from units one and two), what do you consider your own spiritual needs to be?

Small Group Session

Spiritual needs have been largely ignored by nurses because they are seldom as apparent as physical needs. Patients rarely ask a nurse outright to meet their spiritual needs, but sometimes they give loud clues which we fail to hear. Spiritual needs are usually expressed quietly and are often masked by physical or emotional symptoms. The following three case studies provide an opportunity for the group to observe patients and identify their spiritual needs.

Using the scripts provided on the following pages, role play each situation. You will need a narrator, a nurse and a patient for each case study. After each role-play discuss the following questions:

1/How does the patient exhibit or express difficulties in the area of love and relatedness?

2/What seems to give meaning and purpose to the patient's life?

3/In what ways does the patient demonstrate or express a need for forgiveness?

4/What seems to be the patient's concept of God?

5/How meaningful does the patient's relationship with God seem to be?

Case Study: Mr. Rogers

Mr. Rogers is a sixty-eight-year-old black, retired businessman with congestive heart disease and acute respiratory distress. He is married, has several married children who have moved away from town and is an Episcopalian. He has a private room. The nurse in this interaction has cared for Mr. Rogers for two days prior to this conversation. Both of those days he appeared comfortable, cheerful and showed little evidence of any respiratory distress. Both days, however, the night nurse reported that she expected him to "code" at any time. Each night he became short of breath, panicky and demanding, requiring inhalation therapy treatments. After the night nurse had reported a particularly restless night, the nurse has just entered Mr. Rogers's room to do morning care:

Ns1: How do you feel today, Mr. Rogers?

Pt1: Really good!

Ns2: If only your nights were as good as your days. . . .

Pt2: Oh, last night I slept good!

Ns3: Mrs. Simon, the night nurse, said you needed an extra treatment.

Pt3: Oh, well, I missed one during the evening. I had visitors and asked the therapist to come back later. Then I had a little trouble breathing and called for her. [He called for her at 2:00 A.M.]

Ns4: I'd think it would be frightening to not be able to catch your breath. . . .

Pt4: It is. But I'm not afraid to die. A couple of days ago I dreamed that I was close to death—and I really was, they told me—and I saw beautiful scenery. It was so peaceful; I liked it. Now I'm not afraid. If you believe the Bible and are saved, you're okay. I called my priest and he came from St. James Episcopal Church. Then the Episcopal priest from the parish near the hospital came too.

Ns5: Do you feel you're dying?

Pt5: Well, if I do it's okay. I believe in the life hereafter. I was in the hospital in South Carolina a couple of months ago for a hernia. The rooms only cost $45 a day and everybody got a private room. My doctor there knew Dr. Gunther [his present M.D.]; they were classmates in medical school. Isn't it a small world?

Ns6: That must have made you feel at home. . . . [pause] Would you like your bed made now?

Pt6: Yes [turns on TV and appears to concentrate intensely on the program].

Case Study: Mr. Washington

Mr. Washington is a seventy-seven-year-old man with metastatic carcinoma. He has been in and out of the hospital for three months. Discharged three times during that period he has always been readmitted within a week of discharge. Last time he was home for only two days when he became unconscious. He has a wife and brother at home, no children. He is now conscious but lethargic. The nurse in the interaction has stopped into his room on afternoon rounds.

Ns1:   How are you doing today, Mr. Washington?

Pt1:   I'm ready to call it quits.

Ns2:   You feel like giving up. . . .

Pt2:   Yes. I'm ready to die [stares at wall and changes position].

Ns3:   What is the hardest thing for you?

Pt3:   The hardest thing is just waiting and suffering. I can't eat or do anything. I just lie here in the hospital. I fought it for a long time. My wife needs me and I tried to hang on for her sake, but I can't anymore. She works and my brother works. They can make it on their combined incomes, I think. I know it sounds awful to say it, but I want to die.

Ns4:   Sometimes it helps to talk about it.

Pt4:   Yes, sometimes it does [stares at wall in silence].

Ns5:   What do you think it is like to die?

Pt5:   Do you want me to tell you what I believe about the hereafter?

Ns6:   If you want to. . . .

Pt6:   I don't know. . . . Perhaps there's nothing [fidgets]. I am really afraid to die, but I want to be rid of this suffering.

At this point there is a loud interruption from the patient in the next bed who has come back into the room during the middle of the conversation. He admonishes Mr. Washington to "keep fighting" and says, "All the great men in the Bible fought for life . . . Moses . . . Abraham . . . because God only allows fighters in heaven." Then he leaves the room. Mr. Washington appears angry and exhausted.

Pt7:   Well, some men are strong; they can fight; others are weak. I'm weak. I'm tired of fighting.

Ns7:   Mr. Washington, would you like for me to pray with you?

Pt8:   I'm not a Christian. I was brought up in church and I went on Sundays, but I don't want to go running to God now. It's not fair of me. I've ignored God up till now. But please pray in your own way wherever your sanctuary is, not here.

Ns8:   What would you like for me to pray for?

Pt9:   My soul. Just pray for me, Walter G. Washington.

Case Study: Miss King

Miss King is a fifty-seven-year-old woman who lives alone. She has had recurrent dizziness for about twenty years. Her present onset of dizziness, which happened in a beauty parlor, left her depressed and humiliated. She was brought to the hospital by ambulance with her hair still wet. She is still concerned that her hair "looks so terrible." She is being prepared for discharge in a few days. A social worker had been to see her just before the nurse entered the room.

Ns1:   How did the talk with the social worker go?

Pt1:   Well, I'll be getting a housekeeper for four hours a day. She'll keep the house and fix me hot meals.

Ns2:   How do you feel about that?

Pt2:   Well, I don't like it. You can't trust those people. A friend of mine had one and all she did was sit in front of the TV because the housekeeper did everything for her. She got so wrapped up in the TV that one time I went to visit her and she told me to be quiet so she could watch her program. I never went back. I don't want to be like that.

Ns3:   What do you want to be like?

Pt3:   I'm a joiner. I like to be doing things all the time. I have a card-playing group and a shopping group and a group I go to church with. I helped plan the church bazaar. We never really planned anything, but meeting was fun because we were all together.

Ns4:   And you're afraid you won't be able to go places with your friends anymore.

Pt4:   I haven't been able to since I quit work two years ago. And after all I've done for other people. . . . I always remembered my nieces' and nephews' birthdays and graduations. I've been a very generous person. But they don't have time for an old maid aunt.

Ns5:   Does your family know you're in the hospital?

Pt5:   No, they wouldn't care [begins to sob]. I don't want to bother them. Besides, I wouldn't want them to know how sick I am.

Ns6:   How sick are you?

Pt6:   I always have this fear of getting dizzy. I can't go near the stove. It isn't safe, so I can't cook my meals. I'm very sick. I'll end up in an institution eventually. I just pray to God he'll heal me.

Unit 4
Spiritual Needs and the Nursing Process
Individual Exercise
Prerequisite reading: Chapter four, *Spiritual Care: The Nurse's Role*

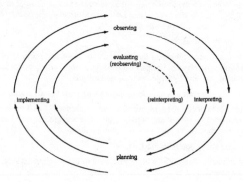

S piritual needs must be recognized and met in the context of the nursing process. The nursing process (see above figure) is the orderly means of assessing a patient's needs and planning care so the nurse can provide optimal intervention.

The objective for this unit is to enable you to enter into the nursing process from the spiritual aspect in four nursing situations. The following instructions for self-study apply to case studies I-IV on pages 24-28. A sample case study is included on pages 23-24.

Part A: Introduction to the Patient
1/Read the paragraph introducing the case study and underline facts that might be clues to spiritual needs.
2/Record in the space provided on the right side of the page (a) the reason you consider the clue significant, and (b) your plans for clarifying or interpreting each clue.

Part B: Nurse-Patient Interaction
In the space provided to the right of each interaction:
3/Evaluate how appropriate and effective the nurse was in interpreting and clarifying observations (remember, not all nursing actions may be helpful).
4/List the spiritual needs which seem to be present.
5/Determine how you would follow up this interaction if you were the nurse.

Sample Case Study: Part A

Mary Clancy is a twenty-four-year-old unmarried woman. She is scheduled for a breast biopsy in the morning. She has no visitors. After the nurse completed her preoperative teaching, the patient began weeping.

① Afraid of how this will affect her future chances of marriage? Allow her to verbalize re: meaning and purpose.

② Breast biopsy - could be cancer, could create fear of death or disfigurement. This, too, might affect patient's sense of meaning and purpose in life - encourage verbalization about surgery.

③ No visitors - are patient's needs for love and relatedness being met? Does she have friends + family? Do they know she is hospitalized? Find out why she has no visitors.

④ Weeping - could be from fear, guilt or totally unrelated to surgery - encourage verbalization.

Sample Case Study: Part B

Ns1: Do you have any more questions about the surgery? Are you worried about it?

an assumption which may or may not be accurate - could have cut off verbalization if too far off base.

Pt1: Well, the doctor said I was going to be okay. He said it seemed to be benign. I'll be all right. I just get a little emotional sometimes.

Ns2: What if it weren't benign... if it were malignant?

Good! The nurse has heard with her "third ear" and expressed what the patient was dwelling on, but was afraid to express.

Pt2: Well, I've had nightmares about that. In fact, when I first discovered it I waited a week before I even went to see the doctor. It was so painful I decided I'd better not wait any longer... so I made an appointment. I guess tomorrow it'll all be over... in the meantime it really... it's unbearable.

Spiritual needs:

Ns3: What seems to be the hardest thing?

① Altered meaning and purpose in life is a possibility.

Pt3: Well, I guess I don't know what I'd do if I had cancer. I believe in God. I've always trusted him for my future. I guess I'm really mad at myself for not trusting him more right now. I was just so embarrassed I didn't tell anyone at church that I was going to have surgery on my breast. I wish they knew now so that they could be praying for me.

② Guilt over what she perceives as lack of faith - needs forgiveness.

③ Need for fellowship with others who would pray - need for love + relatedness.

Ns4: It's kind of lonely. Would it help if I prayed with you right now?

Good - an attempt to meet need #3.

Pt4: Oh! Would you please?

Ns5: Sure. Let's pray. Heavenly Father, thank you that you understand Mary's fears right now. Thank you, too, that you love her and you're going through surgery with her . . . that you're going to be holding her hand as she's there. We pray that you give the doctors wisdom and just give Mary a good night's sleep tonight . . . and just calm her fears. In Jesus' name we pray. Amen.

Pt5: Thank you.

Ns6: Sure.

Prayer picks up on expressed needs for God's forgiveness (e.g. "you understand") and for love & relatedness ("you will go with her"), but does not deal with fear of malignancy and changed lifestyle. It might be good to talk about that after the prayer, when rapport is established.

Case Study I: Part A

Randy Jenkins is an eighteen-year-old college freshman with sickle cell anemia. He is an avid reader. His bedside table has held an assortment of novels, news magazines, liberal arts textbooks, Bibles and devotional material. He has been friendly and outgoing until today. He has pulled his curtain halfway around his bed and is sitting in a chair with a *Time* magazine in his lap, staring at his feet and looking depressed.

Case Study I: Part B

Ns1: You seem kind of down today, Randy.

Pt1: Oh, I'll be okay.

Ns2: What seems to be the trouble?

Pt2: It's the same old thing, I'll learn to live with it, but some times I wonder what's the use . . .

Ns3: You seem pretty discouraged . . .

Pt3: Exam week starts today and here I am, right where I was last exam week. I'll never finish college this way. I'm planning on going into seminary when I get through. I'm sure God is calling me to be a pastor. I'm a lay evangelist in my church now and I'm sure God is calling me into the ministry. But according to all the statistics I probably won't even live long enough to finish college . . . kind of fruitless, isn't it.

Ns4: Would it help if I prayed with you?

Pt4: Hey, that would be great!

Ns5: Father, you know how discouraged Randy is. Sometimes the things you call us to do just don't make sense, and it's frustrating. Thank you, Lord, that you are using Randy in ministry and preparing him to further serve you. Encourage him, Lord. Strengthen him and enable him to continue to sense your purpose and direction in his life. In Jesus' name. Amen.

Pt5: [tears in eyes] It's great to know God cares. Sometimes I forget. I guess that's why I get so depressed.

Case Study II: Part A

Mrs. Greenberg is a forty-eight-year-old woman with metastatic carcinoma of the colon. She has refused palliative surgery to decompress the bowel. She has hired private duty nurses around the clock and fired them in rapid succession. Her husband requested the medicine nurse to "give her a shot that will put her out of her misery forever." Mrs. Greenberg requested a psychiatric consultation this morning.

Case Study II: Part B

Ns1: Mrs. Greenberg, the psychiatrist, Dr. Kirk, called to say he'd be in to see you tonight.

Pt1: Well, he'd better get here. I think I'm going crazy!

Ns2: You're pretty upset . . .

Pt2: You'd better believe I am! You would be too if you were dying and all you had were imbeciles to take care of you! The only reason the doctors want to cut up on me is to get all of my money. Look, I'm dying. Why can't they just leave me alone? I'm not going to sign that permit! . . .

I tried to get nurses and nobody would ever come, so I hired private duty nurses and they're driving me crazy. . . .

My husband doesn't know how to treat me anymore since they discovered my cancer had spread—he treats me like a sick dog—kicks me in a corner. He doesn't even talk to me anymore, except in baby talk. . . .

Nurse, I was a good person. Why does God treat me like this?

Case Study III: Part A

Mary Palmer is a thirty-five-year-old woman scheduled for open heart surgery in the morning. She has been in the hospital for three months. She was unable to work for eight months prior to admission. She has no living relatives. Her housemate moved to Alaska last month, leaving Mary without a home. In discussing her surgery Mary often repeated, "I know I can't live without it, but I'm afraid I'll die on the operating table." For the last week she has spent several hours each day crying. She has developed a good relationship with the head nurse, who has frequently prayed with Mary.

Today, as the nurse's aide was prepping Mary for surgery, Mary began to cry. The aide finished prepping her quickly, then went to the head nurse saying, "You'd better go see Mary right away. She's really depressed!"

The head nurse went in to see Mary, who was sitting in her bed wrapped in a sheet looking out the window. She was dry-eyed, but looked like she had been crying.

Case Study III: Part B

Ns1: Well, Mary, tomorrow is your big day!

Pt1: Yeah, the aide was just in to shave me. She'll be back in a little bit to take me for my shower [gazes out the window as if deep in other thoughts].

Ns2: Are you looking forward to getting outside again?

Pt2: Yeah . . . looks as though I missed the summer, though. It's going to be cold soon, isn't it? I really am anxious to get out though . . . that is if I make it off the table . . . and I'll have to have all those tubes and the breathing machine in . . . I'm really going to hate that.

Ns3: It's kind of scary, isn't it?

Pt3: I really wasn't even scared until fifteen minutes ago.

Ns4: Did something happen then?

Pt4: I guess it hit me then . . . [visitors enter to see patient in next bed, they are loud and overly attentive to the woman they come to visit]. That woman drives me crazy! She has so many visitors and all she does is complain. My friends don't even call, much less visit. . . . I guess I forget, though, that they work. Everybody works except for me. I just lay here. But I have been praying . . . I've been praying a lot. Where's that aide? I really want my shower now!

Ns5: Would you like for me to pray with you now?

Pt5: Right now I'm itchy because of the soap and the hair. Can you pray later?

Ns6: I'll come back at 3:30 when I get off from work and pray with you then.

Pt6: Okay, good. But if I'm asleep, don't wake me up.

Ns7: Okay, but if I don't see you today, I'll come up and see you in ICU tomorrow.

Pt7: They don't allow visitors in ICU, do they?

Ns8: They let nurses in.

Pt8: I won't be able to talk then, but . . . pray for me. Really, don't leave without praying for me.

Ns9: It's a deal.

Pt9: This shower is really going to be something, isn't it! Ever since I've been in the hospital I've had to wash at the bedside . . . and now, you expect me to stand up and balance myself and wash all at the same time. How am I going to wash my hair and hold on? I guess I'm ready to give it a try though.

Case Study IV: Part A

Mr. Jones is a fifty-two-year-old man with ulcerative colitis. He has been constantly surrounded by visitors who seem cheerful and helpful. He appears to appreciate their presence. He continues to have severe diarrhea with little relief from medication. Mr. Jones is a deacon in his church. His pastor visited him yesterday. After that visit he remarked to the nurse about how much he appreciated seeing his pastor since they were good friends.

Case Study IV: Part B

Ns1: How are things going, Mr. Jones?

Pt1: Oh, kind of tired . . . had a lot of visitors today.

Ns2: You do seem to have a lot of friends.

Pt2: They don't really care about me. I've only been here 3 days. They'll stop coming in about a week.

Ns3: Do you think they're pretty helpful to you?

Pt3: Ah, they're pests! They're always hovering around and preaching to me.

Ns4: Would you rather they didn't come at all to visit you here?

Pt4: Well, I don't know. I guess I do want them to come, but I wish I had the guts to tell them off sometime. I'm always Mr. Niceguy and it's tearing my insides up.

Small Group Session

This session provides an opportunity to share observations and plans using the same case studies completed in the individual exercise. For each case study:

1/*Read part A* of the case study aloud in the group (starting with case study I on p. 24).

a/What clues to spiritual needs did you observe?

b/How would you proceed to clarify and interpret each clue?

2/*Role play part B* (starting on p. 24), reading from the scripts.

a/How effective was the nurse in interpreting the patient's environment, affect, attitude and verbal responses?

b/What spiritual needs seem to be present?

c/What would you do to follow up this interaction if you were the nurse? Give your rationale.

3/*Read part C* of each case study aloud to the group (starting below on this page). Each case is analyzed by the nurse involved in the interaction. These are not necessarily the only "right" answers, but are given as examples of responsible nursing action. You may want to discuss how you would do things differently.

Leader's Notes

Next week the group will not meet as usual. Before you conclude this session, read the introduction to unit five's small group session. Divide into *pairs* at the end of this session in preparation for next week.

Be sure to reconfirm the date with the hospital chaplain for session six. Give the chaplain a copy of the questions on the role of the clergy from page 43.

Sample Case Study: Part C

The nurse was sensitive to the fact that Mary was upset about something and was willing to deal with the problem. She might have left Mary more open to respond if she had said, "You seem upset" or "Is something worrying you?" rather than assuming surgery was the cause. Mary's response was a rather unsuccessful attempt to cover her feelings. The nurse accurately "heard" the nonverbal message and expressed the fearful possibility: "what if . . ." Mary then felt free to explain her fears, which encompassed the spiritual needs of (1) meaning and purpose, (2) forgiveness, and (3) love and relatedness.

The nurse moved in to meet these needs through her prayer, thus establishing an open relationship between God, the patient and herself. A close rapport was established. After the prayer the nurse decided to discuss the needs Mary had expressed. She began by asking, "You said that you don't know what you'd do if you had cancer. Sounds like you've been thinking about that lately."

Case Study I: Part C

When Randy poured out his feelings of discouragement and confusion to the nurse, she felt as overwhelmed as he did. She prayed with him to meet her own need—to counteract her feeling of helplessness—but it also met Randy's superficial need at the moment. If she had encouraged Randy to verbalize more of his feelings before she prayed, the nurse might have communicated to him more human care as well as God's care. The prayer served as a Band-Aid to help Randy's mood momentarily, but in the long run it caused him to repress his negative feelings rather than express them.

220

The nurse's goals after the incident were personal rather than patient-care oriented. Randy was discharged the next day. The nurse decided to seriously confront her own feelings about death and life in the face of imminent death. She realized that she identified more closely with Randy's feeling of "what's the use?" than with his hope in God's plan for his future. She made plans to attend a workshop on death and dying. She also began to consider carefully how she would feel and act if she knew she only had several years to live.

Case Study II: Part C

The nurse sensed that Mrs. Greenberg's anger was deeper than dissatisfaction with hospital personnel. She had a hunch that Mrs. Greenberg had requested the psychiatric consultation primarily because she wanted to talk to someone who would listen to her. Neither her husband nor her private duty nurses would allow her to talk about her impending death. Initially the nurse's goal was to be a listener so that Mrs. Greenberg could verbalize. Then her goal became more specific: to assist Mrs. Greenberg to talk about her own death and its meaning to her. She replied to Mrs. Greenberg's tirade by asking, "What is it like to be dying?"

Mrs. Greenberg's anger turned into an expression of *loneliness* and *fear*. She felt abandoned. After listening to Mrs. Greenberg verbalize until she had nothing more to say, the nurse offered to pray with her. She held Mrs. Greenberg's hand to communicate caring and prayed, relating to God the fears, anger and frustration Mrs. Greenberg had expressed, and asking God to comfort Mrs. Greenberg. Mrs. Greenberg grasped the nurse's hand tightly and wept for several minutes while the nurse sat silently with her.

Later Mr. Greenberg stopped the nurse in the hall and asked, "Are you the nurse who prayed with my wife?" She answered affirmatively and he replied, "Well, you have done more for her than anyone she's ever talked to. Thank you."

Mrs. Greenberg's attitude and behavior changed considerably. She was more relaxed and able to talk with her husband and her nurses. She did not fire any more of her private duty nurses. She asked the nurse who prayed with her to pray with her again soon before she died. She died peacefully.

Case Study III: Part C

The nurse responded to the urgency in the aide's request rather than assessing Mary's needs as she entered the room. Mary was still covered with dried soap and hair after being prepped. She was itchy and sticky and anxious about taking a shower for the first time since she was admitted to the hospital. The nurse had previously assessed that Mary had a strong need for *love and relatedness* as well as a need for *meaning and purpose* in life. The aide's report about Mary's depression caused the nurse to immediately assume that spiritual intervention was needed at this point. Mary desperately wanted and needed spiritual support and encouragement; her immediate need, however, was to proceed with the shower. Her physical discomfort and anxiety over the shower were her primary focus. The nurse could have quickly assessed Mary's immediate needs if she had approached her in the first stage of the nursing process—observation—rather than jumping into intervention based on a previous plan.

The nurse's insensitivity to immediate needs thwarted her plan to meet Mary's ultimate needs. But she also demonstrated some good insights. (1) She knew Mary needed her and insisted on sticking with her, in spite of apparent rejection. She had read that patients who have no one to "wait" for them after surgery often do not recover. Mary had already expressed the fear that she would die on the operating table. The nurse had made a mental note that the patients on her unit scheduled for open heart surgery who expressed such fears usually fulfilled their premonition. (2) The nurse was able to see through Mary's rejection of her as a temporary problem; she did not take the rejection personally. She could have been more effective, however, had she seen the rejection as a clue that she was not meeting Mary's present need rather than ignoring the rejection.

The nurse did visit Mary in ICU daily until Mary was transferred back to the floor. She made good postoperative progress and was discharged three weeks later in good health.

Case Study IV: Part C

The nurse noticed the discrepancy between Mr. Jones's pleasant disposition and his disease process, which was giving him increased trouble. She questioned whether the presence of many visitors was really a strong support system or an annoyance. Her statement was nonthreatening and could be interpreted any way Mr. Jones wanted. Mr. Jones chose to use it as an opportunity to express his anger.

This interaction does not leave us with a clearly defined spiritual need, but it does give us a strong clue about the patient's spiritual concerns. Suppressed anger is often a symptom of guilt. Mr. Jones's statement that his friends "preached" and "hovered" also seemed to indicate that he felt guilty around them. The nurse decided to continue to encourage Mr. Jones to verbalize his feelings to determine if he had a need for *forgiveness*.

After several days Mr. Jones alluded to "something terrible" he had done, after which his physical symptoms had first appeared. Since he had already mentioned his good relationship with his pastor, the nurse asked him if he felt that discussing it with the pastor would help. He agreed and called him.

The pastor visited in response to Mr. Jones's call. He was able to confess to the pastor that ten years before he had been unfaithful to his wife. He had never told anyone about the incident but attempted to make up for it by being a loving husband, loyal friend and dedicated volunteer in many church activities. He had been a hard worker and never complained.

The act of confession enabled Mr. Jones to understand God's forgiveness more fully and eventually he could begin to forgive himself. His condition gradually improved.

Unit 5
Use of Self/Use of Prayer
Individual Exercise
Prerequisite reading: Chapters five and six, *Spiritual Care: The Nurse's Role*

The use of self and the use of prayer are closely related. The use of self enables us to communicate in depth with another human being. Prayer is communication with God. Only after we have adequately heard a patient and empathize with his concerns can we pray appropriately for that patient. This unit will help you explore what you have to offer patients from your own personal resources as you exercise the therapeutic use of self. A second objective is to help you communicate with God about your own needs and the needs of patients you may be caring for.

Use of Self
If we are to use ourselves therapeutically with patients, we must be aware of who we are and what we have to offer. We can begin to understand ourselves by considering our strengths and weaknesses.

1/List your strengths and weaknesses, as you see them, on the chart on page 32. Use only the left-hand columns.

2/Strengths and weaknesses are often related. What we experience as a strength at one point may prove to be our downfall at another. On the other hand, the weaknesses we perceive may often be strengths as well.

Look at your lists of strengths and weaknesses. In the right-hand column list how each strength could be a potential problem and how each weakness could be seen as a strength. For example:

Strength: *Leadership ability*	*Sometimes I have difficulty being a follower.*
Weakness: *Stubbornness*	*persistence*

Strengths:

Weaknesses:

3/Review your list of strengths and weaknesses, and consider which ones affect your nursing practice. Circle the two most important ones. Using the charts on this page and the next, examine how these two characteristics can become nursing resources. For example:

Strength/Weakness: *function sensitively and competently with people who seem to need me, but become angry and depressed when people reject or manipulate me.*

How My Nursing Practice Is Affected: *I find that I spend more time with patients who respond positively to me and less time with those who are negative toward me.*

Alternatives: *1) Concentrate time with patients I enjoy and feel effective with.*
2) Concentrate time with patients who frustrate me in order to learn how to be helpful to them.
3) Spend equal time with all patients.

Conclusion: *I am probably more effective with the patients I enjoy, but the others need emotional and spiritual support as well. However, if I concentrate my time with the frustrating patients, I'll probably get depressed and won't be as effective on the whole. Therefore, I'll continue to spend most of my time with patients with whom I have rapport, and also work intensively with one "difficult" patient at a time. I'll write up verbatims of frustrating encounters and analyze them to see how I could have been more sensitive and understanding.*

Strength/Weakness:

How My Nursing Practice Is Affected:

Alternatives:

Conclusion:

Strength/Weakness:

How My Nursing Practice Is Affected:

Alternatives:

Conclusion:

Use of Prayer

4/Prayer is an intimate conversation in a love relationship with God. Have you ever written a letter to God? In a love relationship you share what you are thinking, feeling and dreaming. Whether those thoughts, feelings and dreams are positive or negative, healthy or unhealthy, God cares and wants us to talk to him about them. Express what is going on inside you right now by writing a letter to God.

Dear God,

5/Prayer with a patient can be therapeutic when we articulate to God the feelings and needs the patient has expressed to us. Choose three patients you have cared for recently and write down how you would pray for them based on what you know of their needs. You may want to actually pray as you write.

Patient A:

Patient B:

Patient C:

Small Group Session

T he use of self and the use of prayer with patients usually occur on a one-to-one basis. This session provides an opportunity for group members to practice those skills by interviewing and praying for another member of the group. The structure of the session differs from previous small group sessions. You will meet this week not as a group but in pairs. Every person should choose a partner. The partners should decide on a time when they can spend two uninterrupted hours together to complete this exercise. Reconvene as a group for session six.

Use of Self

(Read with your partner) The use of self involves listening, empathy, vulnerability, humility and commitment. In giving spiritual care the use of self can be facilitated by asking questions which free a patient to discuss spiritual concerns. An evaluation of the strength and meaning of a patient's religious practices can prove valuable in assisting him or her to establish and/or maintain a dynamic, personal relationship with God. A nurse may then intervene more specifically at the patient's level of faith and understanding.

In the following exercise you will each have an opportunity to be both patient and nurse. You should be able to experience something of what a patient feels when asked questions dealing with personal beliefs and religious practices. This exercise should also help you gain confidence in initiating discussion about spiritual needs with patients. You will also get to know yourselves better as you articulate what you believe.

1/Interview each other using the questionnaire on pages 37-38. Complete the entire questionnaire with the same interviewer/interviewee, then switch roles. As nurse, don't be concerned about writing down what the patient says word-for-word. It is more important that you listen carefully and interpret the meaning of the patient's verbalizations.

2/After you have completed both interviews, summarize in writing, in your own words, what your partner has told you. Use the summary questions on page 39.

3/Share your summaries with each other and ask one another:

a/How accurately did you feel I heard what you said?

b/Was anything misinterpreted?

c/Did I seem to understand the feelings you expressed?

d/Did you feel supported during the interview?

e/Were you feeling emotions which you did not express verbally? Was I able to discern them through your nonverbal communication and interpret them accurately? If so, how did that make you feel?

(Read with your partner) On the basis of what you have shared with each other from your interviews and summaries, pray aloud for each other, using the principles from the text about praying for patients. This exercise should help you experience a patient's feelings when prayed for by a nurse. You should also be better able to articulate a patient's thoughts and feelings in prayer and to evaluate your own effectiveness and sensitivity as an empathetic listener. After praying, ask one another:

4/Did you feel I accurately relayed your thoughts and feelings to God?

5/Was there something else you would have liked included in the prayer or anything you would rather I had not said?

6/How did it make you feel when I prayed for you?

Interview Guide

1/What does religion mean to you? _____

_____

2/How does God work in your life? _____

_____

3/How would you describe God? _____

_____

4/Are there any religious practices that are important to you? If so, would you tell me about them?

_____

_____

5/Has being sick (or having problems) ever made any difference in your feelings about God? In the practice of your faith?

_____

_____

6/What about your religious faith is most important to you *right now?* _____

_____

7/Are you dealing with a crisis or illness at this time? If so, could you tell me about it?_____

_____

8/What helps you most when you feel afraid or need help? _____

_____

9/What kind of spiritual support has been helpful to you in the past? _____

_____

10/What is your source of strength right now? _____

_____

_____

11/How can I help you in carrying out your religious practices or in your relationship with God?

_____

_____

_____

12/If you were hospitalized, would you appreciate a visit from your pastor? _____

_____

Notes:

Summary of Interview

1/To what extent is the person you interviewed involved in religious faith? How would you sum up his or her beliefs?

_____

_____

_____

_____

2/How meaningful are the person's religious practices? Do they serve as resources for faith? Do they assist him in his relationship with God? Do they affect his or her daily life?

_____

_____

_____

_____

3/What are the person's sources of hope and strength? Are they founded on reality?

_____

_____

_____

_____

4/What kinds of spiritual support or assistance would be helpful to the person?

_____

_____

_____

Unit 6
Use of Scripture/Referral to Clergy
Individual Exercise
Prerequisite reading: Chapters seven and eight, *Spiritual Care: The Nurse's Role*

S cripture is the authoritative revelation of God. The clergy represent the authority of the church. Both are resources for spiritual care. This unit should enable you to explore the resources of Scripture for both personal and professional use, and help you discover the resources available through your hospital chaplain.

Use of Scripture
In most cases the Scripture portion which will be helpful to your patient will be that which has been meaningful to you.

1/List your favorite Bible verses or passages. Why is each one significant to you? Under what circumstances would it be appropriate to share each passage with a patient?

Verses	Why Significant	Appropriate Use

2/The passages below have been encouraging to patients. Look up each passage and consider situations in which it might be appropriate. Put a check mark in the columns which apply. Mark the passages which are particularly meaningful to you and add any notes you might want for future reference.

	loneliness	guilt	feeling rejected	fear of death	chronic illness	suffering	fear of unknown	Notes:
Deuteronomy 7:6-9								
Nehemiah 9:17								
Psalm 4								
Psalm 13								
Psalm 16								
Psalm 23								
Psalm 32								
Psalm 51								
Psalm 61								
Psalm 116								
Psalm 139								
Isaiah 30:15, 18								
Isaiah 61:1-3								
Matthew 11:28-30								
John 11:25-26								
John 14:1-7								
Romans 8:1-4								
Romans 8:26-28								
Romans 8:38-39								
Philippians 4:4-7								
Hebrews 4:15-16								
Hebrews 13:5-6								
1 John 1:8-9								

Referral to Clergy
(Optional: Include this section if a chaplain will attend the small group session.)
Interview your hospital chaplain using this questionnaire:
3/What functions does the chaplain's department perform in this hospital?

4/How are patients informed of services provided?

5/How can nurses help you?

Small Group Session

T he purpose of the session is to improve the ability of group members to use Scripture as a resource for spiritual care and to understand how the hospital chaplain sees himself as a resource to patients and nurses.

Use of Scripture (30 minutes)

1/Share the lists you have made of favorite Bible passages and explain to the group why each is important. (Have a member of the group compile the lists and reasons for their selection on a chalkboard, overhead transparency or large sheet of paper.) What reasons are most often cited? What principles can be gleaned from your own experiences that apply to using Scripture meaningfully with a patient?

2/Has anyone ever read or recited Scripture to you on a one-to-one basis? How did it make you feel? If it made you feel uncomfortable or angry, what factors made it affect you negatively? If it brought you comfort or joy, what factors contributed to its positive effect?

Referral to Clergy (30 minutes)

The group leader can introduce the second part of the session by saying that nurses and the clergy should be able to work together as a team, meeting the spiritual needs of patients. Open communication facilitates teamwork. Introduce the chaplain to your group. If you have given the chaplain a copy of the questions, he may wish to respond to each of them and then open the meeting up for questions or comments. The group leader could also use the questions to interview the chaplain, or group members could ask him questions from the workbook and others they feel are important. Clarify the format with the chaplain prior to the meeting.

Group Interview with Chaplain

3/How would you describe your ministry to patients?

4/Who else provides services to patients through the chaplain's department (for example, volunteers, local clergy, student chaplains)? What is their role? How does it differ from yours?

5/What kind of spiritual assistance do you think hospitalized patients need?

6/If you had unlimited personnel, finances and facilities available to you, what would you see as the ideal plan of ministering to patients?

7/Have you worked with nurses as part of the health-care team? Has that been a positive or negative experience? What has contributed to making it a good experience? What made it a negative experience?

8/How do you think working relationships can be improved between nurses and clergy?

9/How do you understand the nurse's role in spiritual care with patients?

Leader's Note
Choose two people to present their verbatims to the group next week. Have them photocopy their work for each person in the group.

Unit 7
Utilizing Our Resources
Individual Exercise
Prerequisite reading: Review chapters three through eight, *Spiritual Care: The Nurse's Role*

At this point in the course you should be able to recognize spiritual needs of your patients. You should also be able to include the spiritual dimension in the nursing process and have a firm grasp of resources available to you when giving spiritual care. You are ready to put theory into practice. Peer review and evaluation provide an opportunity for you to grow in your ability to give responsible nursing care. The verbatim assigned in this unit provides a basis for personal review of your nursing practice as an independent study. In the small group session you will receive peer review as you analyze your studies together. Although preparing a verbatim is tedious and time-consuming, you will find it invaluable. Hopefully, you will not stop with the one verbatim assigned but will periodically use this as a tool for personal evaluation.

This unit provides an opportunity for you to analyze your ability to utilize the principles of spiritual care with a patient you have cared for recently.

Utilizing Our Resources
The true test of our skill in the use of nursing resources can only come in the clinical area. The verbatim is a tool which enables us to evaluate ourselves by putting in writing what we and the patient have done and said. Record a verbatim of any patient interaction you have had in which you dealt with spiritual needs. The guidelines below give you a uniform format. You may want to review the verbatims in units three and four of this workbook and chapter four of the text, the verbatim and case study analysis of "Mr. Smith."

1/Background information. Summarize pertinent information from the patient's chart or kardex. Describe the situation, the patient and the context of this interaction.

2/Observations. Describe the patient's immediate environment. Note the appearance of the patient, for example, posture, gestures, affect, attitude, mannerisms.

3/Interview. Enter only direct quotations (as closely as you can remember them) preceded by the initial of the one speaking: Pt for patient, Ns for nurse. If the conversation is too long to record conveniently, indicate summaries of deleted portions in brackets. Number your paragraphs to facilitate easy reference. For example:

Ns1: Hi! I'm Miss Jones. I'll be your nurse today.

Pt1: You're new, aren't you? (eyes darting back and forth) I hope you know what you're doing!

Ns2: You seem worried...

4/Evaluation.

a/*Analysis* of what took place. Note such things as association of ideas, repetition and implications. State insights you gained and interpretations that occur to you.

b/*Criticism* of your own responses. Where did you do well? What could you have done better? What did you learn about yourself in this interaction?

c/*Spiritual needs.* Does the patient seem to be expressing needs you did not pick up while in the situation? How did your own religious presuppositions affect your ability to intervene?

d/*Planning.* What will be your next step?

Small Group Session

The use of case studies and verbatims as a basis for group discussion can be an excellent learning tool. In this session, two people will present their verbatims and evaluations, having provided copies of the verbatim for each group member. (If time permits, the ideal situation would be to have each person in the group present a verbatim. If possible, schedule additional sessions. You may also want to extend this course into another semester and have a Spiritual Needs Seminar for those who complete this course and want to continue to learn from one another by presenting weekly verbatims for group discussion.) The discussion of each verbatim should take 30 minutes and should be based on these directions:

1/The presenter reads the patient's background information and his own observations.

2/The interview section of the verbatim is role-played by two group members. The presenter may want to take the part of the nurse.

3/The presenter reads the evaluation of the verbatim to the group, including the presenter's analysis of what took place, criticism of personal responses, perceived spiritual needs and plans for follow-up.

4/The group discusses the verbatim using these guidelines:

a/Identify any spiritual needs which seem present.

b/Evaluate how effectively the presenter interpreted the patient's environment, affect, attitude and verbal responses, based on the patient-nurse dialog and evaluation.

c/Discuss why you agree or disagree with the presenter's evaluation of the patient interaction.

d/Discuss what you would do next if this were your patient.

Leader's Note

At the conclusion of this session, distribute copies of "Tried and True" (Job in the Today's English Version) to each group member. Encourage them to start their individual work on unit eight immediately. It will take at least three hours to complete the individual exercise, and they will need to pace their time.

Unit 8
Putting It All Together
Individual Exercise
Prerequisite reading: Job (Today's English Version)

The use of a verbatim enabled you to evaluate your spiritual care in an actual patient situation. A case study provides an opportunity to look at the whole picture and plan care accordingly. The book of Job, in the Old Testament, gives us a case study of a man struck by overwhelming loss and physical suffering while in the prime of life.

The objective of this unit is to enable you to review and apply your knowledge of spiritual needs, the nursing process and the use of nursing resources for spiritual care.

Read the book of Job, preferably in a modern translation such as the Today's English Version (available through the American Bible Society). Consider Job (as he is presented in chapters 1—37) to be your patient. The guidelines below will enable you to assess, interpret, plan, implement and evaluate. Allow at least three hours for this study. After skimming through the following questions, you may want to read Job in one sitting, making notes in the margins as you read. Pace yourself during the week to complete all the sections. They will provide the basis for the small group discussion.

Job's Nursing History (chapters 1—37)

Patient's Name   Age   Sex

Place of Residence   Marital Status

Number of Children   Children's State of Health

Occupation   Religion

Physical Status:

Psychosocial Status:

Affect (note changes):

Self-image:

Family dynamic:

Economic status:

Housing/living arrangements:

Significant others:

Attitude toward illness:

Spiritual Status:

Concept of God (note changes):

Source of hope (note changes):

Concept of death and afterlife (note changes):

Use of prayer:

Religious practices he has found meaningful:

Interpretation of Data:
1/What needs can be discerned from the nursing history?
a/physical:

b/psychosocial/spiritual:

2/What needs does Job express verbally?

3/What help has already been given? How effective was it? Why or why not?

Planning Care:
Establish priorities in meeting Job's needs. Then construct a nursing care plan using the format used in your hospital (or the one provided on the next page if no format is available to you).

Nursing Care Plan

Objective _____

_____

Chapter/Verse	Job's Problems	Nursing Approach

Implementing Care:

1/You are Job's nurse and have just heard what he said in chapters 16 and 17. Compose a prayer for Job that would express his needs to God.

2/Would you share Scripture with Job at this point? If so, which passage? Why? If not, what is your rationale?

Evaluating Care:
Read Job 38—42.
1/How did God answer Job (38:1—41:34)?

2/What effect did God's answer have on Job (42:1-6)?

3/How did God evaluate Job's behavior during his illness (42:7-17)?

4/How did God evaluate the help Job's friends gave him during his illness (42:7-17)? What was untruthful about what they had said?

5/What effect did suffering have on Job's life?

What did he learn about God?

What did he learn about himself?

6/Why do you think God allowed Job to suffer?

7/Evaluate the care you have planned for Job. Does it work toward the same goals as the ones God seems to have had for Job? If not, what would you change to bring your plan into conformity with God's plan?

Small Group Session

Preparing a case study on the same patient and comparing observations and interpretations can be a helpful evaluation tool. This small group session is a team conference on Job, bringing together the insights gained from individual work. This conference should help you include spiritual care to a greater degree when planning care for patients and conducting or contributing to team conferences in the clinical areas where you work.

1/Ask someone in the group to present their nursing history of Job. Allow time for other group members to contribute their observations and discuss points for clarification.

2/Ask someone else to summarize the needs of the patient from the nursing history. Encourage other group members to expand the list of needs or question the validity of needs listed by other members of the group.

3/Job expressed three needs verbally—what are they? (See 6:14, 28-29; 13:4-5; 16:3-6; 17:11-12; 19:23; 21:1-2; 16:21; 17:3.)

4/With all the problems Job had, why do you think he asked for these particular things?

5/What kind of care has Job already received? How effective was it? What did his friends do that might have been helpful? How was their intervention unhelpful?

6/Establish priorities for meeting Job's needs. Then write up a nursing care plan for him using the following format (use a chalkboard or other visual aid):

Patient problems	Nursing approach

Unit 9
Personal Resources/Evaluating
Individual Exercise
Prerequisite reading: Chapter nine, *Spiritual Care: The Nurse's Role*

We cannot give away what we do not ourselves possess. Nurses are also physically, psychosocially and spiritually integrated beings who need to experience harmony with God, themselves individually and others. We must draw on the same resources we offer patients—ourselves, prayer, Scripture, and the fellowship of the body of Christ, including the clergy.

The objective of this unit is to enable you to explore your personal spiritual resources and to write up a plan so you can utilize these resources more fully.

Resources
Our personal spiritual resources are the same resources we offer to patients.

1/*The use of self.* One resource within ourselves is our past experience with personal suffering. Reflecting on those experiences can produce growth in our understanding of our own selves as well as the suffering of our patients.

What was the most painful experience in your life?

In what ways was the experience destructive?

In what ways was it constructive?

What did you learn about yourself from the experience?

What did you learn about other people?

What did you learn about God?

2/*The use of prayer.* Has prayer been a resource to you in your daily life? In what ways?

3/*The use of Scripture.* What have you learned about God from Scripture? How is that a resource to you?

4/*The clergy.* In what ways has your pastor or hospital chaplain been a personal resource to you? How could you better utilize the resources of the clergy?

5/*The fellowship of the body of Christ.* Has the fellowship of other Christians been a resource to you? In what ways?

How can you better utilize this resource? (For some ideas see Romans 12; 1 Corinthians 12—13; Galatians 6:1-6; Ephesians 4; and Colossians 3:12-17.)

Values
A nurse's value system, derived from a personal philosophy of life and from beliefs about God and human nature, is the chief determinant of the way a nurse functions. A nurse's personal spiritual resources help to establish and maintain a value system.

6/List, in order of priority, your main goals in life:

7/How do you *actually* spend your time? Fill in the chart below according to what you did last week. Block out time spent at work, meetings, classes, church activities, planned recreation, study, devotions, watching TV, reading, and so on.

	Sunday	Monday	Tuesday	Wednesday	Thursday	Friday	Saturday
5am 6							
7 8							
9 10							
11 12							
1pm 2							
3 4							
5 6							
7 8							
9 10							
11 12							
1am 2							
3 4							

Does the way you spent your time last week demonstrate that you are working toward your main goals in life?

According to your chart, which values seem to be reflected in the way you spend your time? What is most important to you?

Goals

Often our real values are not reflected in the way we spend our time. We may honestly hold very strong beliefs and values, but because we do not plan our time we are overtaken by the seemingly urgent demands around us.

We are each physically, psychosocially and spiritually integrated beings. If one area of our being is neglected, other areas suffer. Planning is necessary to maintain health and to accomplish the goals we have set for ourselves.

Here are some areas to consider in setting your personal goals.

8/*Physical.*
Weight. Is it appropriate for my height and bone structure? If not, what do I plan to do about it?

Grooming. Am I happy with the way I look? If not, what changes do I need to make? When?

Sleep. Do I get enough? too much?

Exercise. What? How often?

Diet. Is it balanced? Are meals regular?

Routine medical and dental examinations. Do I need to make any appointments now?

9/*Psychosocial.*
Supportive relationships. Who are they? How much time do I need with them? What plans do I need to make to maintain them?

Socialization. Am I spending time with persons of different ages, sexes, interests? Do I need to plan in some diversity?

Hobbies—personal and group. Am I developing interests which could be continued if I were disabled? Do I need a hobby?

Cultural enrichment. Am I developing an appreciation for art and music? Am I taking advantage of opportunities in my area? Do I know the history and points of interest in my area? Do I know about other peoples and parts of the world?

Community involvement. Am I aware of important issues in politics? What am I doing to make my community a better place to live in?

Professional growth. What areas do I need to learn more about? What journals should I subscribe to and read? What continuing education programs should I attend? What professional organizations should I join and support?

Intellectual stimulation. What goals do I need to set for reading, television viewing, courses and lectures, interchange of ideas?

Relaxation. What kinds of activities are relaxing to me? How much time do I need to "do nothing"? Have I balanced tension-producing activities in my schedule with relaxation? List the activities you have planned which make you tense; then plan some form of relaxation to follow them:

10/*Spiritual.*
Personal prayer and Bible study. How often? When? What time of day? What should I study?

Prayer partner. Who can I share and pray with on a regular basis? Plan a time to get together.

Small group fellowship. Do I need this kind of fellowship with other nurses? couples? co-ed singles? people in my neighborhood? Which groups am I already involved with? Do I need to cut down on the number of groups I belong to? change to another type of group? become more involved?

Church affiliation. How am I involved already? Am I using my gifts and talents as I should? How can I get to know people better and participate more fully in the life of my church?

Small Group Session

This final session focuses on evaluation. You begin with yourself. But you will also spend time evaluating your small group and, based on this, make plans for the future.

Personal Resources
1/Describe your personal support system (for example, What do you do when you feel overwhelmed, upset or depressed? With whom do you share your feelings? How do they help?)
2/Do you feel that your support system is adequate? If not, what kind of support would you like to have?

Evaluating Your Small Group
Hopefully, your small group has been a personal, as well as a professional, resource to you during this course. This could be the last session of the group, or the beginning of something new. Evaluate together the meaningfulness and usefulness of the group before making further plans.
3/How has the group been helpful to you?
4/How has the group been unhelpful?
5/What has been the high point of the group meetings for you?
6/What was the low point? What made it so?

Ongoing support
If your small group has become a support to you, personally or professionally, you may want to continue meeting. Here are some possibilities to consider:
7/Would a nursing-related Bible study series be helpful? (Numerous Bible study guides for nurses are available; see appendix C in the text for ordering information and descriptions.)
8/Would regular discussion of case studies of patients with spiritual needs help you to give more consistent spiritual care? (You could use the guidelines in unit seven as the basis for regular meetings.)
9/Would you like to meet to pray for one another regularly?

The Spiritual Perspectives in Nursing series is sponsored by Nurses Christian Fellowship (NCF), a national ministry which aims to train Christian nursing students and professionals in evangelism, discipleship, missions, and the integration of faith and nursing. NCF also publishes the *Journal of Christian Nursing,* a 32-page quarterly which will help Christian nurses to relate their faith with their profession and to provide spiritual care to their patients. For information about Nurses Christian Fellowship and the *Journal of Christian Nursing,* write 6400 Schroeder Road, P.O. Box 7895, Madison, Wisconsin 53707-7895.